It's Not Just in Your Head

Demystifying the Brain-Body Connection in Medical Illness

Susan B. Trachman, MD

Health Communications, Inc.
Mt. Pleasant, South Carolina

www.hcibooks.com

Library of Congress Cataloging-in-Publication Data
is available through the Library of Congress

©2026 Susan B. Trachman, MD

ISBN-13: 978-07573-2602-8 (Paperback)
ISBN-10: 07573-2602-1 (Paperback)
ISBN-13: 978-07573-2603-5 (ePub)
ISBN-10: 07573-2603-5 (ePub)

All rights reserved. Printed in the United States of America. No part of this publication may be reproduced, stored in a retrieval system, or transmitted in any form or by any means, electronic, mechanical, photocopying, recording, or otherwise, without the written permission of the publisher.

HCI, its logos, and marks are trademarks of Health Communications, Inc.

Publisher: Health Communications, Inc.
       1240 Winnowing Way, Suite 100
       Mt. Pleasant, SC 29466

Cover, illustrations, interior design, and formatting by Larissa Hise Henoch.

Praise for IT'S NOT JUST IN YOUR HEAD

"*It's Not Just in Your Head*, particularly the section entitled 'Your Two Brains,' is phenomenal! It provides a clear and compelling exploration of the brain–gut connection, an area that has long been enigmatic within gastroenterology. Dr. Trachman skillfully translates complex neurogastroenterological concepts into accessible language, grounding her explanations in sound, evidence-based research. Her ability to make the science understandable while maintaining clinical rigor makes this book both informative and reassuring for patients and clinicians alike.

"What truly sets it apart from others is Dr. Trachman's compassionate, patient-centered perspective. Drawing on her extensive expertise in psychosomatic medicine, she gives a voice to individuals with medically unexplained symptoms and functional bowel disorders—patients who are often misunderstood or dismissed. By validating their experiences and integrating the psychological and physiological aspects of gut health, this book offers clarity, credibility, and hope, making it a valuable and worthwhile investment for any patient seeking a deeper understanding and meaningful insight into their condition."

—**Dr. Tonya L. Adams,** board-certified gastroenterologist and physician executive, and former assistant clinical professor of medicine at The George Washington University

"Full disclosure: I am a long-time fan of Susan Trachman, with whom I have collaborated on patient care for over twenty years—a rewarding, educational, and exciting journey. My always high regard for her as a physician and colleague is solidified at stratospheric heights with the publication of *It's Not Just in Your Head*—elucidating, edifying, and riveting reading! This is a landmark book for all of us who focus on the mind–body connection professionally and for the clients we treat. Susan's straightforward and surefooted command of complex topics makes this work important for those with medically unexplained symptoms and for everyone who is a human body. The content, which covers key psychosomatic processes across organ systems, is relevant for all of us, essential to understanding the complex biopsychosocial choreography of being human."

—**Keith Saylor, PhD, ScM,** president and CEO of NeuroScience, Inc., author, researcher, and consultant on *Hoarding: Buried Alive*

"Dr. Trachman has written a very valuable book that will enlighten physicians, patients, and families who are familiar with individuals that have a variety of persistent symptoms that are thought to have a major psychiatric component. In fact, issues in the brain are 'real' and often comorbid with such well delineated medical syndromes. Patients who experience such difficulties are often upset by labelling the issue as 'all in one's head' and are convinced there is something seriously wrong to account for the pain, fatigue, or other bodily mysterious maladies. This important book reviews the data that such illnesses that can be serious or benign as far as mortality and morbidity often have concurrent brain pathology. Dr. Trachman urges physicians to use a biopsychosocial approach to better understand and thereby explain to the patient who is suffering from unexplained symptoms that maybe possible comorbidity that causes such somatic distress despite negative findings in routine evaluations."

—**Thomas N. Wise, MD,** chair emeritus, Department of Psychiatry, Inova Health System, and professor of psychiatry, The George Washington University School of Medicine

*"I am a very strong believer in
listening and learning from others."*
—Ruth Bader Ginsburg

*For all of my patients who allowed
me to listen and learn from them.
I hope this book makes you feel
heard and understood.*

*And for my children, Ben, Emma, Meg, and Levi.
I hope that I've made you proud.*

CONTENTS

ACKNOWLEDGMENTS · ix

INTRODUCTION · 1

SECTION I: New Insights into the Mind-Body Connection · 11

CHAPTER 1:
The Biopsychosocial Model: Why You Should Read This Whole Book · 13

CHAPTER 2:
Alexithymia: When There Are No Words · 25

SECTION II: Cardiovascular Disease · 35

CHAPTER 3:
Your Achy Breaky Heart: The Role of Stress in Heart Disease · 37

CHAPTER 4:
What's Good for the Heart Is Good for the Brain: The Link Between Depression and Heart Disease · 55

SECTION III: Your Two Brains · 71

CHAPTER 5:
Butterflies in Your Stomach and Other Gut Phenomena • 73

CHAPTER 6:
Is Your Stomach Depressed? The Link Between Your Gut and Mood • 95

SECTION IV: Sneaky Diseases and Psychiatric Symptoms • 113

CHAPTER 7:
Can COVID Cause Psychiatric Symptoms? • 115

CHAPTER 8:
Lyme Disease: The Great Imitator • 127

CHAPTER 9:
Epstein-Barr Virus: Not Just the Kissing Disease • 139

SECTION V: Your Brain on Fire • 151

CHAPTER 10:
Inflammation and Brain Function • 153

CHAPTER 11:
When the Body Attacks Itself: The Mysteries of Autoimmune Disorders and Related Phenomena • 171

CHAPTER 12:
When You're Running on Empty: Chronic Fatigue Syndrome • 181

CHAPTER 13:
Living in a Fog of Constant Pain: Fibromyalgia • 193

CHAPTER 14:
Epigenetics: Why Your DNA Is Not Your Destiny • 209

EPILOGUE • 219

REFERENCES • 223

RESOURCES AND FURTHER READING • 241

ABOUT THE AUTHOR • 243

ACKNOWLEDGMENTS

"Writing is an exploration.
You start from nothing and learn as you go."
—E.L. DOCTOROW

When I first conceived the idea for this book, I thought it would be easy. I was comfortable giving presentations in my areas of expertise and had already been published in professional journals. How much harder would it be just to write something longer? Boy, was I wrong—I knew nothing about writing a book! I had to start from the beginning and learn how to create a manuscript, write concisely, and most importantly, write in a manner that would be appreciated by my audience—patients with MUS. Enter Lisa Tener, book coach extraordinaire! Thanks for your kindness, encouragement, and helpful suggestions. This book would not exist without you.

I have had so many supportive mentors along the way, beginning in medical school. Thank you, "Dr. Kent." You may never read this, but your teaching style (though scary) led me on the journey to psychosomatic medicine. Thank you, Dr. Bernie Frankel, my mentor while I was a psychiatry resident at George Washington University. You supported me in my interest in this subspecialty of psychiatry and introduced me to one of my most incredible supporters, Dr. Thomas Wise. Tom took a chance on me as the first psychosomatic fellow accepted from GW. Your wisdom and humor made coming to work each day an adventure, and your constant encouragement allowed me to become the psychiatrist I am today.

Thank you, Emily Murdock Baker, super editor, who helped turn my novice attempt at a book proposal into a work that gained the attention of multiple literary agents. To Stephanie Tade, for your kindness and support in trying to find me a literary home, and to Steve Harris, who helped me cross the finish line and sign with HCI. Thank you, Christine Belleris, for working with me to make my literary dream a reality. I have to pinch myself to remember I really did publish a book.

Publishing a book is one thing; getting your name out in public is another area where I was a babe in the woods. Thanks to the kind folks at Zilker Media, especially Paige Velasquez Budde and Shelby Janner, who started me on my PR journey, and at Trusty Oak, especially Corie Luzon, and my excellent social media guru, Jillian Neuhaus.

I have been so fortunate to have the support of the greatest friends—Ellie Mandel, my BFF, who has been with me since we sat next to each other in Mr. Malinowski's Spanish class. Despite my personal deficits, you still think I'm a hero. To Helen and Steve

Acknowledgments

Kraus, my friends forever, thanks for your generosity, support, and humor. To my book club friends who have listened to my endless updates about this book and cheered me on: Louise Molton, Dr. Robin Merlino, Dr. Ellen Horwath, Chilo Obolensky, Tena Knudsen, and Hannah Craven. Thank you, Dr. Molly Sebastian, for your support and wisdom, and for agreeing to review this manuscript. Dr. Catherine McCarthy, you were an inspiration. Watching you write and publish your book spurred me on in my own publishing journey. Thanks also to Dr. Emma Trachman for her helpful input, especially in the section on autoimmune disorders. Aside from being a wonderful daughter, you are a great doctor in your own right!

Last, but certainly not least, thank you to all of my patients. This book exists because you asked for it, and without your request, I probably wouldn't have pursued this adventure. I hope you and others with MUS find the contents helpful.

INTRODUCTION

*The part can never be well
unless the whole is well.*
—PLATO

Have you ever experienced physical symptoms that have no obvious explanation? Have you visited multiple physicians, including specialists, who order laboratory tests and scans only to tell you, "The results do not explain your symptoms"? Hearing this, have you felt you were not taken seriously? Misunderstood? Shamed? Or even disbelieved? If so, you are not alone. You are in good company with individuals who have "medically unexplained symptoms" (MUS). Ten of the most common problems that lead adult patients to seek help from their primary care physician include chest pain, fatigue, dizziness, headache, swelling, back pain, shortness of breath, insomnia, abdominal pain, and numbness. These account for almost

40 percent of primary care visits, yet a "biological" cause is found only about a quarter of the time.

In this scenario, your doctor may express frustration at the lack of a diagnosis. More importantly, their exasperated response can make you feel disrespected, uncared for, and even hopeless. The medical community has different names for patients with MUS, such as somatisizers, functional disorders, or even malingerers. A study of patients with MUS found that reassurance from a health provider suggesting that negative test results means, "Nothing is wrong," can make you believe your concerns are not taken seriously or are outright rejected.

Lucy's Story

Lucy[1] told me about visiting multiple doctors over several years before one finally arrived at a diagnosis for her symptoms.

She said, "After a week of what seemed like an intense flu with great fatigue and achiness, I felt exhausted. I dragged myself to work as the director of a nonprofit, took one- to two-hour naps at lunch, kept working, and dragged myself home. I slept the rest of the day into the night, woke up tired despite excess sleep, and slept all weekend to recover. I had times of achiness and times of intense pain, particularly when it was humid. When I think about it, though, I remember having a low-grade fever toward the end of the workday for several months before the flu."

Lucy's Experience with the Medical Profession

I asked Lucy about her experience with the medical professionals she visited in search of answers to her troubling symptoms.

---

1   All names have been changed to protect patient privacy.

She replied, "When I sought medical care, I often teared up when describing my symptoms because I would try to soldier through much of the time, and telling the story made the emotions come up. The doctors would then say, 'You're probably depressed. See a psychiatrist, and they can put you on meds.' I knew, however, that this was more than that, and I continued to seek help. Luckily, I'd been seeing a therapist, and she said, 'Well, of course, you feel somewhat depressed—you have no energy, and you're in pain.' She also knew there was more to it and encouraged me to continue working toward an accurate diagnosis. I think she was also the one to identify that it might be chronic fatigue"—a close cousin of fibromyalgia and sometimes considered on the same spectrum.

"How many providers did you consult before arriving at a diagnosis?" I asked.

"Two or three primary care physicians, a couple of specialists at major hospitals that were no help at all, a chiropractor, a nurse, and an osteopath. Finally, I got a diagnosis when I switched to a different primary care physician. She said it was fibromyalgia. But the only thing she had to suggest was a low dose of antidepressants, which might help somewhat but would not address the cause, just relieve symptoms. I talked to some people who were in online fibromyalgia or chronic fatigue groups. They were very resigned to their illnesses, had some side effects from the low-dose meds, and said that as soon as they stopped them, their symptoms returned. So, I knew that wasn't the path for me. I was certain I could heal. I was determined."

Was Her Voice Heard?

I wondered if she felt her providers listened to her concerns during this long process, answered her questions, and made her feel respected.

"Did you feel understood/respected/valued by your providers?" I asked.

"Not by the docs at the hospital," she replied. "They were super dismissive. And I felt they treated me with judgment. They had a superiority complex!"

Sometimes, patients with MUS feel hopeless and worthless after seeking answers from medical providers who are not forthcoming.

"Lucy, how did it make you feel? Did any provider make you feel hopeless, worthless, or unimportant?"

"Absolutely; at least two or three made me feel marginalized and even judged. I had to drag myself to those appointments. I took a cab to one because I had no energy to get there by public transportation. It was demoralizing."

The Toll of Medically Unexplained Symptoms

Finally, I asked, "Did any of the providers you consulted suggest it was all in your head?"

In a very animated fashion, she replied, "Yes!"

For many people, doctors remain figures of authority. Traditionally, doctors are the ones you turn to when you are ill. We have fancy degrees, use expensive instruments, have lots of diplomas on the wall, and often wear white coats, just like the good guys on TV and in movies, where we often play the heroes who swoop in to save the day. So, what happens when the authority tells you, "There's nothing wrong"? You may doubt your feelings, think negatively about yourself, or believe you are weak for feeling like you do. If Lucy's story resonates with you and makes you tear up or become angry, know that you are not alone. There is hope for finding a diagnosis for MUS. As Lucy learned about the role of the brain-body connection and the various sources that contributed to her symptoms, she found relief over time. She sought answers to her questions and did not assume that the answers she was already given were her only options.

In my private practice and academic roles, I have witnessed the toll MUS takes on my patients. It can impact social and professional lives and cause real strain on personal and family relationships. Worse yet, it can cause anxiety and depression or make you feel out of control of your body—experiencing real symptoms that are not easily explained.

Aside from the negative emotional toll, the actual disabilities associated with MUS have an economic cost. Individuals with MUS take more sick leave, have higher unemployment rates, and generate higher healthcare costs due to frequent diagnostic tests and procedures that are not always in their best interest.

"It's All in Your Head"

Most of the medical profession understands the importance of the therapeutic relationship and feels responsible for nurturing it, even when it is difficult. However, many doctors fluctuate in their willingness and capacity to engage with patients who have disorders we cannot readily explain. Physicians often feel overwhelmed and frustrated by the task of caring for patients with medically unexplained symptoms and lack confidence in their ability to meet their patients' needs. As a result, the messages received by patients can sound like, "There is nothing wrong with you. It's all in your head." This was true for Lucy and many other patients arriving in my office. Sometimes the doctor's language can be dismissive or minimize the symptoms. One patient, who had had an undiagnosed blood pressure issue that was making her anxious, was told, "You're just having spells." Other times, patients are told, "Stop using Dr. Google," which is demeaning.

The part of the message that says, "It's all in your head," is true because your brain is in your head. However, many healthcare providers do not explain to their patients with MUS that there is a brain-body connection, and to assume the brain and body function independently is patently wrong. The brain and body are a unit. Think of your brain as the CEO of the company, your body. Each organ system is a manager, and the managers are responsible for sending feedback to the "boss" so that they can adapt to the working environment and adjust as necessary. Whatever your brain is feeling creates repercussions in various parts of your body. The reverse is true as well. If you feel sick to your stomach, your gut sends a message to your brain: "We don't feel well." In turn, your brain responds.

By the time you finish reading *It's Not Just in Your Head: Understanding Medical Illness from a Biopsychosocial Perspective* I hope you will appreciate that, yes, part of your symptoms may very well be in your head. The two-way connection between your brain and your body is constantly active, and sometimes the physical illness you experience results from what is going on in your brain via bidirectional communication.

"Trachman, Diagnosis!"

I have been a psychiatrist for over thirty years and have taught medical students, residents, and postresidency fellows for much of that time. My specialty is psychosomatic medicine. That is a subspecialty within psychiatry that focuses on the brain-body connection and the impact of psychological factors on physical disease. The majority of patients referred to me by other specialists have coexisting medical and psychological illnesses. Often, diagnosing and evaluating the psychiatric component of the patient's complaint leads to an amelioration or even remission of the physical complaint. Sometimes, we even identify unexpected coexisting medical factors that other specialists did not previously consider.

My interest in this area began as a third-year medical student. The chief of my psychosomatic medicine specialty service, Dr. Kent, was a British neurologist and psychiatrist who wore his hair long, his mustache bushy, and clogs as his preferred footwear much of the time. He modeled himself after Mick Jagger of the Rolling Stones and, in his own way, had a rock-star persona. He had a real following among the male psychiatry residents, many of whom tried to imitate his bravado by similarly letting their hair grow long, wearing clogs, and stylishly popping up the collars of their white coats, just as he did. Every morning, we made rounds in one of the major hospitals at the Texas Medical Center in response to requests from any medical services that had questions about an issue regarding patient care that tests or examinations alone could not readily explain. We were the psychiatry *CSI* team.

Dr. Kent could be pretty intimidating. His preferred facial expression was a snarl; he was highly sarcastic and frequently condescending. On rounds in the hospital, he was fond of pointing to a patient who might be walking in the hallway and calling on one of us inexperienced students, demanding, "Diagnosis?" Hesitation in responding—or worse, an incorrect answer—led to cutting remarks, a stare, and a scowl. Once, I got lucky when he picked on me. I had fortunately reviewed the symptoms of Parkinson's disease the night before, and coincidentally, Dr. Kent set his sights on an older gentleman who was shuffling down the hall.

"Trachman, diagnosis?" he demanded.

"Parkinson's?" I answered.

"Are you asking or telling me?" he grunted, obviously dismayed that he didn't get the better of me.

Dr. Kent was not a charmer, but to his credit, he was an excellent teacher. I learned so much about psychiatry and also neurology and internal medicine, necessary information if you want to practice psychosomatic medicine.

By the end of the rotation with Dr. Kent, I planned to apply for a psychiatry residency and hoped for a fellowship in psychosomatic medicine. Just before the end of this elective, I witnessed one of the funniest cases I ever saw in medical school, which sticks with me to this day. It often reminds me not to assume I know the answer to a problem without considering all the possibilities.

We were asked to see Mrs. Plato, a lovely sixty-five-year-old woman who had heart surgery several days before and was being monitored in the intensive care unit (ICU). She had a history of diabetes that intensive care specialists could not control, and they wondered whether they'd been missing a psychological cause for her elevated blood sugar.

Mrs. Plato was in the surgical ICU after her operation as a precaution; her open-heart procedure had gone well. Despite many attempts to control her blood sugar, her readings remained inconsistent with what was expected since she received insulin and was prescribed a diabetic diet in the hospital. After interviewing this very cooperative woman, we learned she had a large family that visited often. She was overweight and understood she would need to comply with a diet prescribed by the American Diabetes Association after discharge.

Her family history included several members with diabetes. She insisted that she took her insulin as prescribed. We reviewed her chart and noted that her blood sugar levels were highest after family visits. We wondered, *Were these visits stressful?* Stress can cause a surge of cortisol or stress hormones, resulting in a higher blood sugar reading. During the interview, she told us she looked forward to her family visits, and they all got along well. Perhaps her excitement about seeing them caused the same result? As it turned out, the family visits were connected to the problem, but not in the way we expected.

Generally, after interviewing the patient, one of our team members would perform a brief physical examination. Occasionally, we detected something that the medical management team hadn't noticed. In this case, to conduct a heart exam, we had to gently elevate her very pendulous breasts. Much to our surprise, we found not a heart issue but a package of Twinkies! Her family brought her treats that she hid under her voluptuous mammary glands. Final diagnosis: elevated blood sugar secondary to Hostess snack foods! I still remember the first and only time I witnessed Dr. Kent laugh after we consulted with the infamous "Twinkie Lady." He was so loud that the nurses could hear him at their station down the hall.

What's Next on Your Journey?

After completing *It's Not Just in Your Head*, you will understand how the brain-body connection is involved in many common medical illnesses, such as heart disease, gastrointestinal disease, infections, and autoimmune disorders. Patient examples throughout illustrate how these disorders can be challenging to diagnose but can be understood in the context of the bidirectional communication between the brain and body. A breakdown of various biological processes will be explained, revealing how these common disorders occur from a physiological standpoint. Reviewing treatment options will help empower you and provide hope for managing your illness and living your best life.

We did not expect to find such a novel answer to our consultation question about Mrs. Plato's elevated blood sugar. But if you assume you already know the answer, you will never consider alternatives. Lucy kept looking until she found alternative solutions to improve her health. Sometimes, searching for answers means looking outside the box. You never know, you might find your own version of a Twinkie.

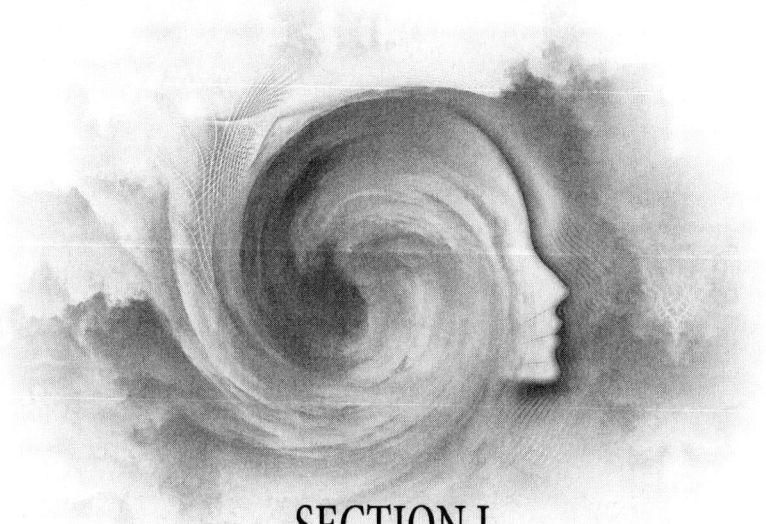

SECTION I

NEW INSIGHTS INTO THE MIND-BODY CONNECTION

CHAPTER 1

THE BIOPSYCHOSOCIAL MODEL: WHY YOU SHOULD READ THIS WHOLE BOOK

Nothing will change unless or until those who control resources have the wisdom to venture off the beaten track of exclusive reliance on biomedicine.
—GEORGE ENGEL

The belief that the mind and body are separate entities makes no sense, right? If I cut off your head, could you continue to live? Of course not! But for centuries, brilliant philosophers and physicians considered the mind and body to be distinct entities. This idea led the medical profession to view illness solely as a biological cause. Expanding on that hypothesis explains why so many individuals find their way to my waiting room. They are told, "There is nothing medical we can find to explain your symptoms. It must be in your head. Go see a psychiatrist." This limited view fails to consider that, as humans, we have thoughts and emotions, and that we live and work in a world where we are impacted by our environment and those around us. As this book discusses, many illnesses are significantly affected by psychological factors such as trauma, as well as social factors.

For example, untreated depression is an independent risk factor for cardiovascular disease. Anxiety can lead to gastrointestinal illness. Stressful home or work environments can initiate or exacerbate the symptoms of autoimmune disorders. To successfully treat these disorders, some early pioneers in medicine conceptualized a more holistic approach to illness management. In the decades that followed, this would evolve into the biopsychosocial model.

Benjamin Rush, considered the father of American psychiatry, firmly believed in the holistic approach to medicine. Many consider him a forerunner in psychosomatic medicine.

Sir William Osler, one of the most famous English physicians of the nineteenth century, believed that the future of medicine should include an understanding of the influence of the mind over the body and their interdependence.

Dr. Helen Flanders Dunbar was a unique woman of her time. She attended Yale Medical School, specializing in medicine and obstetrics, and received her PhD from Columbia University in the 1930s. She founded the American Psychosomatic Society and was an early editor of *Psychosomatic Medicine*. Her book *Emotions and Bodily Changes: A Survey of Literature on Psychosomatic Interrelationships* popularized the term *psychosomatic* and led to the holistic approach to medical practice.

However, in the nineteenth and twentieth centuries, as medicine advanced technologically, greater emphasis was placed on cellular disease mechanisms. When Louis Pasteur and Robert Koch made their discoveries about the role of bacteria in disease, they laid the groundwork for the principle that every disease has a single specific cause. As a result, mental or emotional factors took a less prominent role.

On December 10, 1913, identical twins George and Frank Engel were born in their family's Upper East Side brownstone in New York City. They were delivered by a very prominent physician, who happened to be their paternal uncle. Uncle Manny, known as Dr. Emmanuel Libman-Sacks, was a highly respected physician with an elite clientele. Despite his friendly sounding moniker, Uncle Manny was described as "cold, aloof, and intimidating."

Uncle Manny's office was conveniently located in the brownstone where George and Frank grew up, but it also made for a decidedly nontraditional arrangement for the family. It was not unusual for his famous patients—Albert Einstein, Fanny Brice, or George Gershwin—to arrive at their door waiting to see their renowned physician. His office was in an area of their home considered sacred and not to be breached.

The home was so immersed in medicine that the twins' older brother had several surgeries performed by a world-famous head and neck surgeon in their sterilized bathroom. George recalled, "I thought that was ordinary living, that such medical activities went on in every house." Uncle Manny greatly influenced George and was instrumental in his life's pursuit of understanding the molecular basis of disease.

George's mother had a profound influence on him as well but in a much different way. Mrs. Engel was described as "dramatic" and suffered from multiple physical complaints that were out of proportion to any physical findings. She was diagnosed a "hysteric" because no biological basis could be found for her many physical symptoms. Even her brother Manny, the prominent physician, was at a loss to explain the basis for her numerous disorders.

In modern terms, she most likely had an illness that would be classified as "psychosomatic," a term later made famous by her son. As an adult, George reflected, "She was an influence on my life with which I struggled—that it be my destiny to solve the problems Uncle Manny could not."

As a young boy, George suffered from fainting spells. He recalled fainting after receiving a typhoid shot, which his doctor brushed off and admonished, "It's just a faint." Feeling dismissed, George's embarrassment led him to find elaborate ways to hide the episodes. During his extensive career, he focused on understanding how psychological phenomena could influence physiology.

These principles of Engel's model included the biological, psychological, and social dimensions of an individual's life and the perception that individuals suffer as a whole, not as isolated organs. Physicians, therefore, should have a holistic approach to illness, including the patient's emotional state and environment.

How Is the Biopsychosocial Model of Illness Used Today?

The biopsychosocial model of wellness and medicine examines how the three aspects—biological, psychological, and sociological (BPS)—occupy roles in health and disease. The BPS model stresses the interconnectedness of these factors. Common illnesses such as heart disease and cancer have psychological and sociological components that combine with biology to cause illness. For example, it is estimated that 30 percent of cancers are associated with tobacco use, and diet accounts for a significant proportion of digestive tract cancers. So, the biological factor may be a familial predisposition to cancer, but if you smoke, that risk adds to your genetic loading. Similarly, if your family has a risk for gastrointestinal cancers and you eat a diet high in processed foods, red meat, and sugar, your risk increases overall.

On the other hand, understanding the various psychological and social risk factors for disease can help mitigate your genetic inheritance. For example, heart disease risks are increased by factors such as hypertension, smoking, high cholesterol, and type A personality traits. But as this book demonstrates, interventions can be designed to decrease risk, suggesting strategies for behavioral change. These might include referral to a smoking cessation program, offering suggestions for an anti-inflammatory diet, or enrolling in a regular exercise program.

The BPS model was used to develop new treatment approaches for patients living with chronic pain, which affects approximately 50 million Americans. The cost of treating pain and lost productivity ranges from $70 billion to $100 billion annually.

Traditionally, pain research has focused on sensory modalities, and neurological transmissions were identified solely on a biological level. In other words, the experience of pain was conveyed directly from your skin to your brain without consideration of psychological or social factors. This was called the *reductionist* or *biomedical* view of pain.

Your nervous system is composed of two major parts or subdivisions: the central nervous system (CNS) and the peripheral nervous system (PNS). The CNS includes the brain and spinal cord.

The brain is the body's control center. The PNS is a vast network of nerves linked to the brain and the spinal cord, containing sensory receptors that help process changes in your internal and external environment. The gate control theory of pain was formulated in 1965 by a neurobiologist and a psychologist who proposed that spinal nerves act as gates that allow pain to reach the brain or close these gates and prevent pain messages from getting through.

This theory helped researchers understand how individuals experience different types of pain and develop treatment strategies. So, what influences a person's perception of pain?

- **Emotions.** Negative emotions like anxiety, depression, and chronic stress can increase pain. Once you're in the cycle of depression and pain, for example, it can be challenging to know whether your depression is making your pain worse or whether your pain is worsening your depression. They may influence each other. Therefore, it's essential to acknowledge the link between mental health and chronic pain.
- **Brain disorders.** Your brain is the processing center for pain, so if part of the brain isn't working correctly, you might not process pain in a healthy way. People with schizophrenia, for example, often don't perceive pain in the same way as those without this disorder. This was horrifically illustrated for me when, as a second-year psychiatry resident, I was called to the emergency room to evaluate a young man with a diagnosis of schizophrenia. In a psychotic state, he had mutilated his genitals and arrived in the ER holding them in a bag.
- **Stronger signals.** An old wives' tale suggests that you should rub the affected spot if you hurt yourself. This is an excellent example of "closing the gates" of pain. When your brain

perceives a secondary stronger signal coming in, it doesn't pay as much attention to the first painful signal. My dentist demonstrated this to me one day when I needed a Novocain shot to have her work on my teeth. She was able to give me the shot without causing any pain because she put pressure on the inside of my cheek for a few minutes before inserting the needle loaded with anesthetic. I was amazed at the difference. The sensation of pressure overrode the feeling of the needle entering my skin.

- **Drug use.** Prescription medications, as well as illegal drug use, affect the way your body processes and perceives painful stimuli. Opioids, which are often prescribed for pain, have a strong gate-closing effect—usually. However, the overuse of opioids can cause a rebound effect and lead to increased sensitivity to pain over time.
- **Central sensitization.** People with chronic pain often experience heightened pain responses to nearly everything. If you live with chronic pain daily, your nervous system develops an abnormal response to everyday stimuli. For example, clothing may hurt, and walking may be too painful to bear. In other words, things that seem innocuous and theoretically shouldn't be perceived as painful are the reality for those with conditions like rheumatoid arthritis or fibromyalgia. In these disorders, the body's gates are left wide open, often requiring medical assistance to shut again.
- **History of trauma.** Post-traumatic stress disorder (PTSD) is an anxiety disorder experienced by approximately 30 percent of people who have witnessed or lived through a trauma in which they anticipated extreme bodily harm or death

to themselves or someone they love. Women are twice as likely to develop PTSD compared to men. The highest rates of PTSD are consistently linked to a history of physical and sexual abuse. A 2007 study at the University of North Carolina looked at the role of PTSD and trauma on the health status of women seen in their gynecology clinic who were diagnosed with chronic pelvic pain. The investigators found that almost 50 percent of women in their sample with chronic pelvic pain reported a history of sexual or physical abuse. One out of three women in their sample also had PTSD, indicating a high degree of psychiatric morbidity in this patient population. The investigators recommended obtaining an abuse and trauma history as part of a comprehensive evaluation of patients with pelvic pain.

There are other proven differences in how individuals perceive and respond to pain. Devising a one-size-fits-all approach would not, and does not, work effectively. For example, research from the Centers for Disease Control and Prevention documented that women, individuals from lower socioeconomic backgrounds, military veterans, and people residing in rural areas have a higher prevalence of pain. Studies are mixed regarding ethnic and racial differences, with some reporting the highest rates among non-Hispanic White people. Explanations for racial differences include enhanced physiological pain sensitivity, cultural differences, and reduced access to care. When controlling for income and adverse life events, the differences in prevalence are diminished but not eliminated.

As the biopsychosocial model evolved and spread through the scientific and medical communities, it became increasingly apparent that managing chronic pain through solely biological pathways was a dead end. This new approach offered valuable additional avenues for pain management that diversified the number of treatment providers capable of managing chronic pain and led to breakthrough clinical approaches with better outcomes.

The biological processes contributing to pain influence psychosocial elements such as emotion and cognition. Emotion is the more immediate reaction to an uncomfortable physical sensation like pain. For example, when you mistakenly stub your toe, the first response is something like "*Ouch!*" However, your thoughts or cognitions give meaning to the emotion, such as *Damn, that was stupid!* In some cases, pain-related cognitions can lead to an amplification of the experience of pain.

In another situation, you have a history of cancer, you have been successfully treated, and you are in remission. Suddenly, you feel pain on the left side of your chest, where your surgical scar is a reminder of your previous diagnosis. In this case, the response to pain may be different than when you stubbed your toe. The first response may still be "*Ouch,*" but the cognition may be very different, something like, *Oh no, I hope this doesn't mean the cancer has returned.* This, in turn, may give rise to a cycle of worry, leading to an increased perception of pain.

In these two examples, the *process* of pain is the same. It is the psychosocial factors and *response* to the pain that are different.

The most effective treatments for patients with chronic pain are those that include a BPS approach. Comprehensive treatment of pain, addressing the biopsychosocial aspects of the pain experience, is more clinically effective than conventional medical treatment by itself and more cost-efficient as well. For example, the ability of an individual to return to their prior levels of activity with comprehensive treatment approaches is 65 percent compared with only

35 percent with conventional medical treatment. Patient reports of pain improvement with comprehensive pain treatment are equal to or greater than those reported with the use of traditional medical treatment with opioid medication.

What Would a Biopsychosocial Approach to Pain Management Look Like?

The stepped-care model proposed by the Veterans Health Administration advises initiating care with the least resource-intensive services before progressing to specialty care through a patient-centered, BPS framework. An interdisciplinary approach includes self-care, which might consist of weight loss if appropriate; a healthy lifestyle including exercise, good nutrition, and proper sleep hygiene; and smoking cessation. Additional treatments in such a framework include opioid and nonopioid medications, as well as psychological therapies.

- Exercise is the most recommended self-management strategy, which can improve sleep, facilitate weight loss, stimulate endorphin secretion, and reverse deconditioning.
- The most common psychologically based intervention for chronic pain is cognitive behavioral therapy (CBT), which involves restructuring maladaptive beliefs, attitudes, and behaviors contributing to the disease burden. The theory behind CBT is that if you can change the way you think, you can change the way you respond to what's physically happening in your body. You learn new strategies to manage discomfort by *shifting your focus and perspective*, even if the pain doesn't disappear. A solid therapeutic relationship is crucial for maximizing the effect of CBT, with the best candidates

being motivated, educated individuals with clear-cut goals and coexisting mood or anxiety disorders that tend to amplify pain. A clinical review article examined data on more than fifty-nine studies that included five thousand participants with various types of chronic pain. Investigators found that CBT had a positive, though modest, effect on reducing pain, disability, and distress associated with chronic pain.

- Antidepressants, as well as physical therapy, have been used effectively to relieve chronic pain. Physical therapists who specialize in treating chronic pelvic pain are experts in employing stretching exercises, massage, and pelvic floor training.
- Acceptance and commitment therapy (ACT) is an action-oriented approach to psychotherapy that stems from traditional behavior therapy and CBT. Clients learn to stop avoiding, denying, and struggling with their inner emotions and, instead, accept that these deeper feelings are appropriate responses to certain situations that should not prevent them from moving forward in their lives. With this understanding, clients begin to accept their hardships and commit to making necessary changes in their behavior, regardless of what is going on in their lives and how they feel about it. ACT was developed in the 1980s by psychologist Steven C. Hayes, a professor at the University of Nevada. His theories emerged from his own experience, particularly his history of panic attacks. Eventually, he vowed that he would no longer run from himself. He would accept himself and his experiences.

Lower socioeconomic status (SES) has consistently been associated with every aspect of poorer health, including increased morbidity, decreased life expectancy, and higher infant mortality. Not surprisingly, lower SES is also consistently associated with an increased risk for pain. Research studies report that the prevalence of chronic pain of any origin, as well as that of pain-associated disability, is twice as high in low- and middle-income countries as in high-income countries. One explanation could be that individuals with lower economic status may not have accessible health care, leading to chronic pain as a result of an injury or underlying disease state. However, another explanation may be the association of behavioral factors with lower income. One example of this is obesity, secondary to a diet of processed and fast foods that are readily accessible in the United States and less expensive than healthy alternatives. Increased tobacco use and alcohol use, both of which are risk factors for chronic pain, are also more prevalent in lower-income communities. Finally, living in a more stressful community due to economic hardship and increased crime can contribute to poor sleep. Chronic sleep deprivation is associated with an increase in chronic pain.

Understanding these factors is critical to providing a successful treatment plan for patients with chronic pain. Nutritional education, assessment, and treatment for sleep disturbance, and learning to moderate alcohol use can all help reduce the experience of pain for many patients.

The idea of the mind-body connection is a familiar one. However, as with most ideas or theories, the concept has been modified and elaborated over time. The chapters that follow show how the mind-body connection is in play in many medical illnesses. Wellness is more than simply the absence of disease. It is an active process toward a healthier, happier, and more fulfilling life, including physical, psychological, and social dimensions.

CHAPTER 2

ALEXITHYMIA: WHEN THERE ARE NO WORDS

So runs my dream: but what am I?
An infant crying in the night:
An infant crying for the light:
And with no language but a cry.
—SIR ALFRED, Lord Tennyson

I wrote this book to help you understand how your physical symptoms may not correlate with objective findings or laboratory studies. Instead, these symptoms may result from more than what meets the eye—or the eyes of the medical professional. Because we are more than the sum of our genetic material, psychological and environmental factors can combine with genetic predispositions to cause medical conditions.

But what if you were unable to identify or express your feelings? It might make it challenging to communicate with your healthcare provider, leading to a problem in arriving at the correct diagnosis. The term *alexithymia* derives from Greek and translates to "no words for emotions." Individuals with alexithymia have difficulties identifying, understanding, and expressing emotions. In addition, they may struggle to distinguish between physical sensations and emotional states. As a result, those who experience alexithymia can erroneously attribute physical signs to an illness and may search for a medical explanation when there is no underlying physical cause. For example, a 2021 study of two hundred patients seen in an outpatient internal medicine office with complaints consistent with medically unexplained symptoms showed that almost half qualified for a diagnosis of alexithymia.

If you have alexithymia, you may be viewed as socially awkward or lacking in appropriate emotions for a given situation. If you try to see a therapist about this, you may have difficulty answering some basic questions, such as "How are you feeling today?" because you don't know. The estimate of people with this trait is about 13 percent of the population and is twice as likely in men. It can occur congenitally, from birth, or can be secondary as the result of a brain injury.

People with alexithymia who experience bodily cues such as a racing heart, difficulty breathing, or body pain often cannot identify their origin. Some of these individuals misinterpret the physical components of feelings because they cannot recognize an emotional state and its physical accompaniments. Think about what happens when you laugh uncontrollably at something you find amusing. You know you feel happy or elated, but laughing hard can make you short of breath or create gastrointestinal symptoms. Or what about the saying "I'm laughing so hard, I'll pee my pants." Those of us without alexithymia think nothing of this. However, some people with alexithymia might laugh, not connect the behavior with a feeling of gaiety, and interpret the shortness of breath as a symptom of illness, such as this young lady:

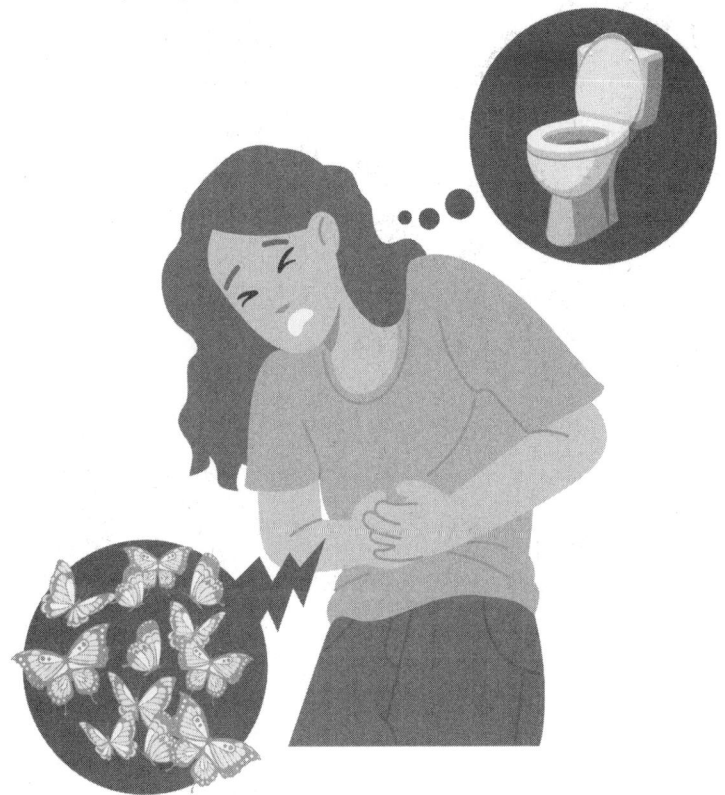

Fig. 2.1 Am I Falling in Love, or Do These Butterflies Mean I Have to Use the Bathroom?

What Causes Alexithymia?

Most researchers believe that primary alexithymia is the combined result of genetics and environment. In one study published in 2018, investigators reported that participants with alexithymia had differences in an area of their left-brain hemisphere compared with their unaffected counterparts. The affected participants had smaller amounts of gray matter in their insula. The insula is crucial in integrating sensory signals with emotional and cognitive processes, particularly those from your body.

In a different study, patients with alexithymia underwent brain imaging while being shown various facial images of angry, sad, and happy individuals and were asked to discriminate between them. The results showed that alexithymia correlates with decreased activation in brain areas associated with emotional awareness while viewing facial expressions.

Sometimes the inability to identify or express emotion comes from cultural differences. For example, in many Asian cultures, mental illness is stigmatizing; it is considered to reflect poorly on family lineage and can influence others' beliefs about the suitability of an individual for marriage. It is more acceptable for psychological distress to be expressed through the body than through the mind. One researcher who described the presentation of psychiatric illness among a group of Chinese patients reported that the resemblance to alexithymia was striking.

Some authors suggest that alexithymia can develop as a reaction to an acute and severe traumatic event or in the presence of early life stress. A majority of studies demonstrate the coexistence of early life stress and alexithymia in patients with mood disorders. A survey completed in young adult German volunteers diagnosed with alexithymia found that early neglect rather than physical or emotional abuse was most highly correlated with severe forms of alexithymia. The authors defined early neglect as "the experience of a caretaker's failure to provide adequate affection and emotional support for the child."

According to a 2011 study, people who experience adversity in childhood tend to have difficulty identifying their emotions. A Portuguese study published in 2023 sought to identify and analyze the relationship between adverse childhood experiences (ACEs) and alexithymia in adulthood. In agreement with earlier research, the authors reported that, in their sample, there was a statistically significant positive correlation between childhood emotional neglect and difficulty identifying and distinguishing feelings from bodily sensations.

Andrew

I saw Andrew, a twenty-eight-year-old graduate student, as part of a forensic evaluation. Aside from my clinical practice, I consult with attorneys and organizations regarding claims of psychological damage. In this case, Andrew was suing a pharmaceutical company for what he said were damages he suffered as the result of taking a prescribed acne medication ten years earlier. The attorneys representing the pharmaceutical firm wanted me to evaluate his claims to see if they were valid.

When he walked into my office, I was struck by how tall, thin, and pale Andrew was. He walked to one of the chairs, slumped down into it, and spread out his long legs.

"Are you comfortable?" I asked.

"As much as I can be with all of the pain I have," he snorted. His pain was not isolated to one area of his body but was everywhere.

I thought, *This is going to be a long evaluation.* And it was. Andrew and I spent the next three hours reviewing his history and how he came to my office. He told me he lived with daily pain and had been experiencing it more or less constantly for ten years. Despite this, he completed his undergraduate education at a highly competitive university and was enrolled as a doctoral student at another major university.

"How has your life been impacted by the pain you experience?" I asked.

"My life has been highly compromised by the pain I suffer daily. I can't compete in some of the athletic activities I once enjoyed. I can't even sit comfortably in this chair," he replied. "As a result, I have to make accommodations regarding the classes I select and the physical positions I have to contort into so that I can study."

Andrew told me about the significant stressors he was experiencing. As we dug deeper into his history, he said his mother was always overly involved in his life and frequently called or emailed him to offer medical suggestions. She insisted on knowing the results of his multiple medical consultations and searched the internet to find alternative treatments for him. Andrew had seen many medical specialists since he began on this decade-long journey and had endured exhaustive testing and imaging studies. Despite this, no definitive reason for his pain could be found.

I asked him if he ever felt angry or resentful about losing the ability to enjoy some of his hobbies and activities.

He replied, "I do miss some of them [activities], but no, I don't feel angry or resentful."

He also denied ever feeling depressed. Andrew experienced an increase in the intensity of his pain when he left home for college, and he said it seemed to worsen after he experienced a loss or disappointment. For example, when he was denied a desirable teaching appointment, he claimed he felt disappointed but not angry. However, his symptoms worsened.

His symptoms also increased in intensity after a highly charged interpersonal event, but he failed to recognize that during these times he was very angry. For example, when he argued with his mother on the telephone, his perception of pain increased. Andrew told me, "I've tried to correlate the stress in my life and the pain. . . . I just can't." This was also the case when I asked him to try to do so in my office.

Andrew agreed to testing provided by a psychologist at a renowned pain clinic as part of his overall evaluation. The results indicated he had traits consistent with alexithymia.

Andrew's experience with chronic pain, which he attributed to exposure to acne medication, proved to be a medical mystery. Despite numerous evaluations, all his test results were normal. Nevertheless, it had become very burdensome to his quality of life and was the basis of his lawsuit.

A significant body of research links chronic pain, such as Andrew reported, to symptom amplification and attribution theory. *Symptom amplifiction* is the conscious or subconscious behavioral pattern where an individual's subjective reports of symptoms are inconsistent with their known impairment. In the context of alexithymia, *attribution theory* explains how these individuals struggle with the impact of their lack of emotional awareness on their interpretation of symptoms. Therefore, when a symptom occurs, their thought process attributes causality to a physical cause rather than internal emotional reactions they cannot identify.

Chronic pain, in this case, refers to pain that persists or progresses over time and is often resistant to medical treatments. In research studies on chronic pain, alexithymia is frequently reported in patients with the most severe forms of physical distress. A possible explanation can be found in the multidimensional nature of pain. One aspect of pain is *affective*, which is the unpleasant experience of pain. The other is *sensory*, which refers to the intensity of pain. The studies that account for this distinction found a specific association between alexithymia and the affective dimension of pain in patients like Andrew likely because the affective dimension of pain comes from a particular brain structure, which also regulates and processes emotions.

Not surprisingly, Andrew lost his lawsuit. No evidence could connect his report of pain to any fault on the part of the drug manufacturers who made his acne medication. I did not treat him because of the nature of my involvement in this case. Most likely his physical complaints reflected the multiple stressors he was enduring. However, due to his alexithymia, he could not make the connection between his emotions and his physical symptoms.

How Does Alexithymia Lead to Amplification of Physical Symptoms?

Symptom magnification also includes the tendency to report physical symptoms in an intense and disturbing way. Research suggests that alexithymia can be associated with the amplification of physical symptoms like those Andrew reported. Because people like Andrew struggle to identify and express emotions adequately, they can misinterpret bodily sensations related to emotion, like a rapid heart rate when they are scared or excited. Instead, they overemphasize the physical sensation and believe it is due to a medical disease or condition. Rather than identifying an emotion as the cause of the physical symptoms, they often focus on the symptoms themselves, which can heighten the perceived intensity, and is one of the reasons they can frequently be diagnosed with a medically unexplained condition.

How Does Alexithymia Impact Medical Conditions?

An early theory suggested that people with alexithymia have difficulty regulating negative emotions—because they don't recognize them—which leads to altered immune system activity. Studies that examined patients with alexithymia and their immune status reported that they generally have less robust immune systems.

Another theory suggests that people with alexithymia have alterations in their autonomic nervous system, the part of the nervous system that is not under voluntary control. This includes body functions such as breathing, heart rate, and blood pressure. Support for this theory is from studies that show some people with alexithymia have increased resting cardiovascular activity, like increased blood pressure and heart rate.

Does alexithymia lead to unhealthy habits that impact medical illness? The inability to identify emotions or have difficulty with regulation can lead to poorer choices in nutrition, substance abuse, or other behaviors that act to decrease the negative feelings. For example, alexithymia is elevated in people with eating disorders, excessive gambling, and alcohol abuse. Additionally, some studies of alexithymia showed that these individuals have worse overall nutrition and lead a more sedentary lifestyle, which contributes to the onset of disease.

Alexithymia is associated with cardiovascular diseases and is a predictor of cardiovascular risk in healthy people. In addition, alexithymia is a risk factor for early death after a heart attack.

There is limited research on ways to treat people with alexithymia because of their limitations in understanding and expressing emotions. However, a study to evaluate the benefits of group psychotherapy in twenty patients who survived an acute myocardial infarction showed a significant improvement in alexithymia after four months with one ninety-minute session per week compared with an educational treatment focused on cardiovascular risk factors. The group psychotherapy included several techniques, such as progressive relaxation and role-playing, communicating emotions nonverbally, describing their dreams to others verbally or in written form, and painting their interior feelings. Patients were further asked to apply these techniques in their daily lives. The educational group received information about cardiac risk factors.

Unfortunately, because alexithymia patients have difficulty recognizing emotions and their link to physical symptoms, they may delay seeking help, leading to a worse prognosis. Traditional psychiatric interventions such as psychotherapy and medication are not usually successful. The best approach is CBT, which has succeeded in some research studies. However, because of their difficulties communicating their feelings, alexithymia patients find it challenging to build and maintain close relationships with others and to appropriately use social support to protect themselves from the potentially pathological influences of stressful events.

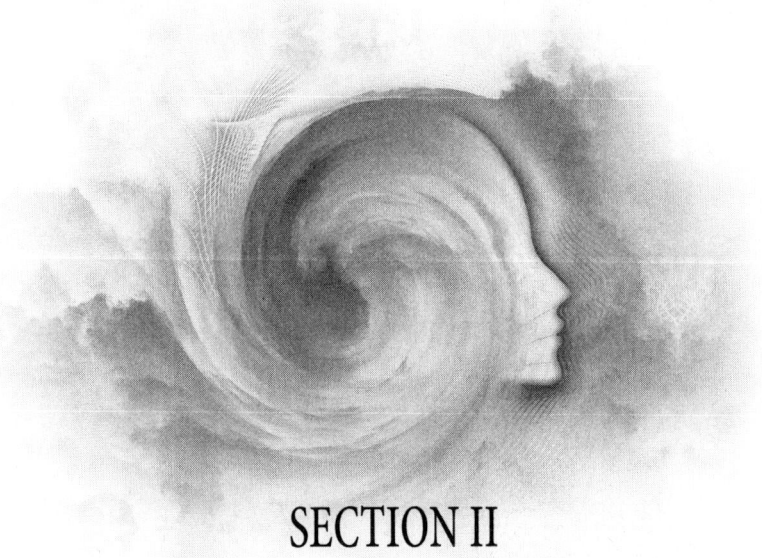

SECTION II

• • •

CARDIOVASCULAR DISEASE

CHAPTER 3

YOUR ACHY BREAKY HEART: THE ROLE OF STRESS IN HEART DISEASE

I will never have a heart attack.
I give them.
—GEORGE STEINBRENNER, former owner, New York Yankees

On December 27, 2016, actress Carrie Fisher, of *Star Wars* fame, died at the age of sixty—four days after suffering a massive heart attack. Her mother, Debbie Reynolds, who was expecting her for Christmas dinner, died of a stroke the following day.

When musician June Carter Cash died of complications from heart surgery in 2003, no one was more devastated than Johnny Cash, her husband of many decades. When Johnny was hospitalized four months later to manage his diabetes, his condition was poor but not poor enough to account for his death solely based on this disease.

Mary Tamm was beloved in Britain for her role in the television show *Dr. Who*. In 2012, she died of cancer. Just hours after delivering the eulogy at his wife's funeral, her husband, Marcus Ringrose, described as "fit and well," died while sitting at his computer, writing thank-you notes to those who sent their condolences.

Maybe you know someone who has lived through a similar situation. What explains the sudden onset of a heart disorder after a significant stressor or loss of a loved one? The answer is stress cardiomyopathy, also known as Takotsubo's cardiomyopathy. In this condition, intense emotional or physical stress causes rapid and severe heart muscle weakness. It can occur following a variety of emotional stressors, such as grief, fear, or severe anger. It can also happen following numerous physical stressors to the body, such as a stroke, a seizure, difficulty breathing, or significant bleeding. Stress-induced heart disease has even been reported after a vigorous Zumba class.

Takotsubo's cardiomyopathy was first reported in 1990 in Japan and named after a Japanese octopus trap. The appearance of an affected human heart on an arteriogram resembles an octopus trap. The following photos illustrate images of a female patient with Takotsubo's on the right compared with a photo of a Japanese octopus trap on the left. See the similarity?

In an unaffected individual, the left ventricle, the heart's pumping chamber, contracts and pumps blood normally. In a person suffering from Takotsubo's, the left ventricle has a characteristic ballooning shape during contraction. In addition, the bottom of the heart is enlarged and barely moves.

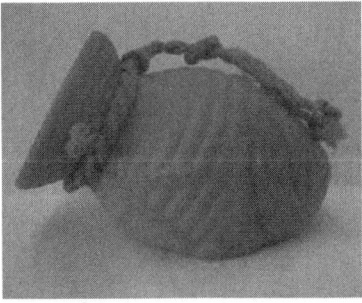 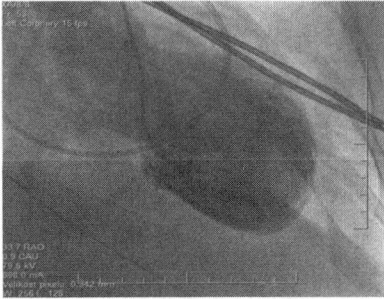

Fig. 3.1 Similarities Between an Octopus Pot and Imaging from a Patient with Takotsubo's Cardiomyopathy

One of the critical risk factors for Takotsubo's cardiomyopathy is being a female in menopause. Estrogen, which acts as a protective hormone against Takotsubo's cardiomyopathy, declines during the years leading up to menopause. Other known risk factors include a history of neurological or psychiatric disorders, such as migraine headaches and seizure disorders, depression, post-traumatic stress disorder, anxiety, work-related stress, poor sleep, acting as a caregiver, and experiencing a disaster. After experiencing significant physical or psychological stress, someone prone to developing Takotsubo's will experience a change in the left ventricle. When you experience a stressful event, your body produces hormones and proteins like adrenaline that help you cope with stress. Your body responds as if it is being threatened. This is commonly known as the *fight-or-flight response*. The result may overwhelm your heart muscle. In addition, excess adrenaline can narrow the small blood vessels that supply your heart, causing a decrease in blood flow. In some cases, the surge of adrenaline can bind to your heart cells, which causes a large calcium intake, limiting those cells from allowing your heart to beat normally. While this situation is dangerous, in most cases, induced cardiomyopathy is temporary and can be reversed.

One-third of patients diagnosed with Takotsubo's have a preexisting psychiatric history, which is an independent risk factor. Some patients with preexisting psychiatric illnesses produce excess amounts of stress hormones, which may put them at risk for a stress-related heart disorder. Some investigators wondered if the poorly controlled psychiatric illness was the reason for this risk factor. This theory has been disproven. The research shows unequivocally that *a direct link exists between the brain and the heart, and a depressed or anxious brain can cause or exacerbate cardiovascular disease.*

In our fast-paced society, it's not uncommon to feel stressed as more and more is demanded of us; work, our daily commute, the financial pressure of making ends meet, and home and family responsibilities can all weigh on us. Add in the stress of national and world events, exacerbated by the near-constant bombardment of this information, and it's no wonder we feel unnerved. Yet the way we process and experience stress varies greatly. It may be influenced by a complex interplay of genetic, biologic, psychological, and social factors. Men and women tend to experience and deal with stress differently. Women are more likely to think and talk about their stress and to reach out to others for support. Men typically respond to stress with distraction, such as engaging in physical activities as an escape. Temperament also impacts our response to stress. For example, during the COVID-19 pandemic, people who identify as introverts appreciated working from home. The forced confinement was not a hardship, and grocery delivery services, first-run movies on streaming services, and a world at a standstill might have seemed like a godsend to those who relish being homebodies.

On the flip side, extroverted people, who thrive on interpersonal interaction and human contact, found the social isolation, monotonous routines, and separation from friends and loved ones burdensome and lonely, which caused a spike in depression and anxiety in people of all ages.

Researchers have proven that stress is a significant cause of cardiovascular disease. To understand how this happens, we must recognize the role of the brain, particularly the part of the brain responsible for emotions: the limbic system.

The amygdala plays a prominent role within the limbic system. It can be thought of as the brain's "emotional coding center." It is a key factor in the body's response to a fight-or-flight situation and is critical for responding appropriately to a stressful situation.

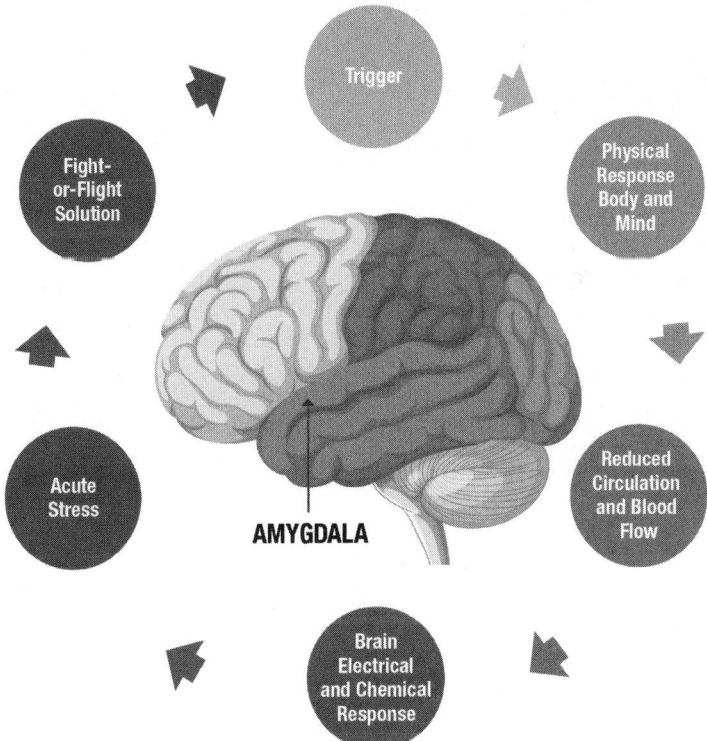

Fig. 3.2 The Amygdala Hijack

This diagram represents the brain and body circuit during a stressful event. Acute stress triggers a fight-or-flight response. Responding to the stress, your body undergoes multiple changes as it reacts to a perceived catastrophe in progress. Your heart rate and blood pressure increase and signal a component of your blood called platelets to release the chemical neuropeptide Y. This can cause your blood vessels to spasm—and can even temporarily block the heart vessels. This effect occurs because in people with preexisting plaque buildup in their coronary vessels, the surge of stress hormones can destabilize or rupture a plaque, leading to formation of a clot. In certain instances, this activation can be adaptive and something that has served humans as a survival mechanism. For example, if you were in extreme danger and needed to escape something—a predator, for instance—an increased heart rate and higher levels of stress hormones would improve the likelihood that you would escape safely.

Now that we no longer need to fear predators—unless, perhaps, you are hiking in the wilderness without your bear whistle—the real danger to this adaptation can come from the repetitive cycle of chronic stress. Prolonged isolation, fear of losing your job, or working in a toxic environment can cause your body to undergo the same physiologic phenomena. Here, the fight-or-flight response is not helpful and can harm you.

Most investigators agree that stress responses arise when demands on individuals exceed their psychosocial resources or adaptive capacity. In a fascinating study at a major hospital system in Boston, researchers measured the amygdala activity of research subjects while at rest. They reported that the volunteers who exhibited increased amygdala activity at rest also had increased inflammation in their blood vessels and a higher risk of cardiovascular events over the next four years. The authors proposed that emotional stress signals a region of the amygdala to activate part of the nervous system, producing inflammatory white blood cells in the bone marrow—our body's response to any kind of assault (infection, injury, or trauma). These changes may contribute to heart attack, stroke, or sudden death. This study was among the first to demonstrate a direct relationship between emotional stressors and the risk of cardiovascular events.

Stress can occur even before you are born. A study published in 2018 examined the effects of prenatal stress on the later development of cardiovascular disease and depression in the offspring of the women studied. The investigators hypothesized that the gender differences in the development of coexisting cardiovascular disease and depression in the offspring (women show persistently higher rates) may, in part, be due to a process that occurs in fetal maturation during the development of their brain, heart, and vascular system. The results of the study reported that prenatal stress and inflammation program the fetal brain to increase the risk for depression and cardiovascular disorders later in adulthood.

A Brief Intermission to Understand the Autonomic Nervous System

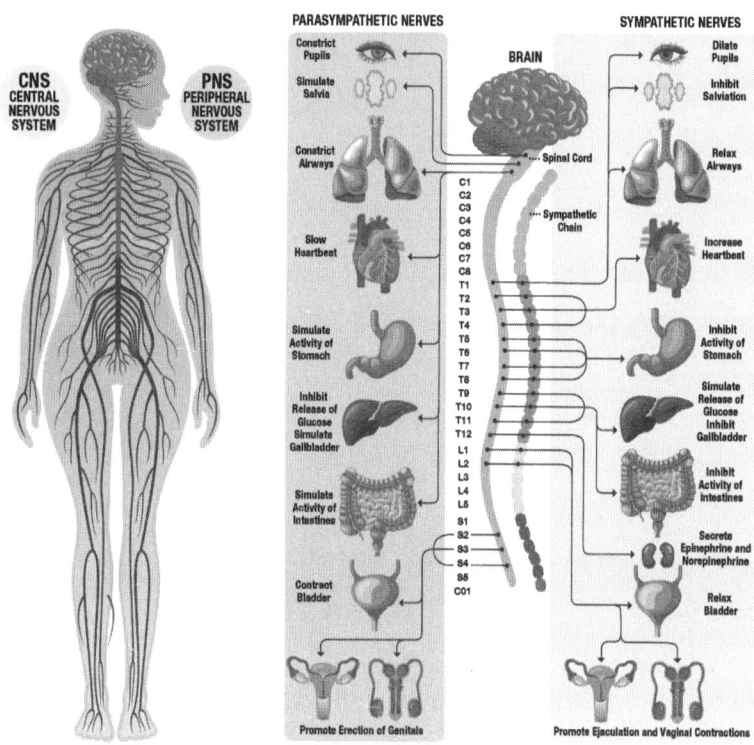

Fig. 3.3 Composition of the Human Nervous System

Before we explore the impact of psychological stressors on the development of hypertension (high blood pressure), we must understand the role of the body's autonomic nervous system. On the one hand, the autonomic nervous system (ANS) regulates the functions of our internal organs, such as the heart, stomach, and intestines. The ANS is part of the peripheral nervous system (as opposed to the central nervous system: the brain and the spinal cord). The ANS also controls some of the muscles within our bodies. It functions involuntarily and reflexively. Therefore, it is not under voluntary control. There are two parts of the ANS: the sympathetic and the parasympathetic nervous systems. In an emergency—like those experienced by combatants, first responders after a disaster, or even emergency room personnel—the sympathetic nervous system is dominant. It increases your heart rate, blood pressure, respiration, and other body functions. The ANS's primary role is to help you survive.

On the other hand, the parasympathetic nervous system is involved in the relaxation process and causes a decrease in respiration, heart rate, and blood pressure. Knowing about these differences has helped clinicians devise treatment options that work on maximizing the role of the parasympathetic nervous system in an effort to manage all types of heart disease, including high blood pressure. Take, for example, my patient Kathy.

When I arrived at my office one morning, I found three messages from a woman named Kathy. I'd never met or worked with her, and she sounded desperate.

"I need help. I can't take this. I know I'm going to die because my blood pressure is sky-high! I've been to the emergency room three times, and they tell me it's stress, but I know it isn't. I've never had high blood pressure before, but now I'm having chest pains. I don't know what to do!" she said in an agitated voice.

Kathy had been referred to me by her gynecologist, whom I know well. Given the panicked nature of her call, I was surprised to learn that my colleague had given Kathy the referral three years earlier. My schedule was pretty full the day I got her message, but I finally had a break long enough to call her back to try to assess the situation. She shared that she was convinced she had heart disease and had already seen her internist, a cardiologist, and three separate emergency room physicians during her frequent visits to the ER. Fortunately, I had a cancellation in my schedule, so I could see her within a few days. She wanted to know what to do in the meantime, but since I was not yet her physician, all I could do was tell her to call her primary care doctor for a limited prescription for an antianxiety medicine. She did so, but her primary care doctor told her to "read a book and relax."

On the day of her appointment, Kathy arrived early and was neatly dressed. She thanked me profusely for getting her in so quickly and immediately began to cry. Trying to alleviate her distress, I suggested she take a few deep breaths and tell me what was going on. Although Kathy was in her sixties, she looked youthful but was also relatively thin. She told me she was so anxious she could not eat and had lost ten pounds in the past month. She added that she could not sleep because she feared waking up with heart palpitations. *Why*, I wondered, *had she waited three years to call me?*

Kathy was a retired government employee married to a man fifteen years her senior. Her parents were deceased, both from cardiovascular-related disorders. Although her husband was elderly, he was physically and mentally healthy. Kathy had no prior history of hypertension or heart disease. She was not a smoker, exercised regularly, and was not overweight. She drank alcohol only occasionally. As she described her history, I made note of the fact she described past episodes of anxiety and depression. She was treated for both, as well as an eating disorder, in her thirties. Several of her family members had been treated for anxiety. Kathy described herself as having a type A personality and felt she was "high-strung."

Kathy's husband complained that she "reacts too strongly" to nonstressful situations. Her behavior was so off-putting to him that he bought a house an hour's drive from their current residence and planned to live there by himself. He agreed to cancel the purchase of the home if she got help. Kathy said that when they both were working full-time, they only saw each other in the evenings and on weekends. Now that they were both retired, they were together 24/7.

Kathy desperately wanted to sell their current home and move. However, she couldn't decide where to live and worried that their house was too small and cluttered. Her husband had just celebrated a milestone birthday, and she was worried that they had only limited time left to enjoy one another. These factors culminated in her feeling "frantic" and a sense of urgency to "do something."

Kathy was experiencing a significant amount of self-imposed stress that had caused her elevated blood pressure readings. In addition, she was having chest pain that was also likely due to stress. When we are stressed, our muscles contract. The chest wall is very muscular and was probably clenching, creating chest pain. On one of her visits to the ER, Kathy was given an antianxiety medication, and the symptoms disappeared within minutes.

Hypertension, or high blood pressure, is often called the "silent killer" because it is possible to have this disorder without any overt symptoms. It is a common condition that affects approximately one-third of Americans and explains almost 40 percent of all deaths due to cardiovascular disease. Hypertension contributes to health disparities, being more common in non-White communities. Beyond the health risks to people, it is also a major contributing factor to healthcare costs. Actuaries project that treatment for hypertension will cost almost $275 billion annually by 2030.

Some risk factors for hypertension are widely recognized. They include obesity, a diet high in fatty or salty foods, a history of tobacco use, chronic sleep disorders, and excess alcohol use. Genetic factors such as a family history of heart disease can be somewhat modifiable with lifestyle changes, but unfortunately we cannot pick our genes. Just like eye color or adult height, they are fixed at birth. Psychosocial stressors affecting heart disease are not as easily identifiable, but since 1900, researchers have made increasingly more sophisticated attempts to do so.

In the 1950s, two cardiologists, Dr. Meyer Friedman and Dr. Ray Rosenman, developed the concept of the Type A personality. They created this concept after observing similar behavior patterns in many of their patients with hypertension. Later, they developed a list of personality traits that are risk factors. They include an intense desire to achieve, a highly competitive drive, a need for recognition in achieving goals, involvement in multiple functions under time restrictions, an accelerated rate of execution of several physical and mental functions, and increased mental and physical alertness. These behavioral characteristics and a sense of time urgency resulted in impatience and hostility. Their patients engaged in excessive speed in eating and walking and displayed intense frustration with ordinary situations such as waiting in lines. Further, they exhibited hostility when driving and had little tolerance for perceived trivial errors in themselves and others. They slept poorly because of anger or frustration and cared little for altruism.

By 1981, evidence for the significant association between Type A behavior and cardiac disease was so strong that the National Heart, Lung, and Blood Institute included Type A behavior among the independent risk factors for cardiovascular disease. Since then, a great deal of research has been published attempting to link this behavior specifically to heart disease. Not all elements of this personality type pose an equally significant risk, however. The most distinctive characteristic associated with Type A behavior is irritability, the most stable predictor of cardiac risk. Many studies have replicated this finding, and this characteristic poses a risk not only for the onset of cardiovascular disease but also for increased death rates among recipients of heart transplants.

If you see yourself in this description and are worried, I can offer you good news. Although a tendency toward low frustration tolerance and irritability may be considered a fixed trait, it is one of many risk factors amenable to modification.

The Good News: Positive Personality Traits Might Decrease Risk

Research regarding the brain and cardiovascular disease has focused on the risk factors for predicting the onset and course of heart disease, including hypertension, stroke, and more recently, dementia. We've reviewed the roles of stress, psychiatric illness, and personality type, as well as psychosocial factors that have adverse effects on the body and can contribute to heart disease. Now let's get to the good side of the ledger.

Positive psychological well-being (PPWB) is a broad concept that includes elements such as life purpose, personal growth, positive emotion, life satisfaction, happiness, and optimism. PPWB reflects the positive feelings, thoughts, and behaviors of individuals who evaluate their lives in a favorable light and generally feel they are functioning well.

Two theoretical approaches characterize research in this area: eudaimonic and hedonic well-being. These terms derive from Aristotle and his theorizing about what constitutes a good life. In more modern terms, *eudaimonic well-being* is understood as fulfilling one's potential and identifying meaningful life pursuits. In contrast, *hedonic well-being* focuses on our pursuit of pleasure and happiness. Where eudaimonic well-being addresses our evaluations of how we function in life, hedonic well-being emphasizes how we evaluate our feelings about life. Some other constructs, such as optimism and vitality, probably fit in either of these categories and have been linked to positive cardiac health as well.

The eudemonic concept contains elements such as

- **Purpose in life.** The extent to which you experience purpose and meaning in your life
- **Personal growth.** The extent to which you seek to realize your full potential and recognize that you are constantly evolving
- **Self-acceptance.** The extent to which you hold favorable views of yourself
- **Environmental mastery.** The extent to which you effectively manage your environment or perceive your life as under your control
- **Autonomy.** The extent to which you act independently without concern for external pressures

The following concepts are categorized under hedonic well-being:

- **Happiness.** The extent to which you consider yourself a happy or unhappy person

- **Satisfaction with life.** The extent to which you judge the overall quality of your life to be satisfactory
- **Positive affect.** The extent to which you experience pleasurable feelings and a lack of depression or anxiety

The relationship between PPWB and cardiovascular disease involves the presence of health-promoting processes and the absence of health-deteriorating processes. Examples of positive or restorative processes would be eating a diet rich in fruits and vegetables, sleeping eight or more hours per night, and engaging in regular exercise. People who possess PPWB have less likelihood of engaging in harmful processes such as smoking and heavy alcohol consumption. Therefore, individuals with these attributes should experience less inflammation in their system than those without them.

Two researchers, Julia Boehm and Laura Kubzansky, reviewed an enormous amount of data that revealed how PPWB protects against heart disease. They found that people who possessed characteristics of eudaimonic well-being were less likely to initiate smoking behavior, and if they were already smokers, they were less likely to continue. The same was true in individuals who possessed traits of optimism and vitality. Moderate use of alcohol was not significantly linked to traits of PPWB, but excessive use was. For example, people who possessed eudaimonic characteristics were less likely to have histories of heavy alcohol use or dependence. Those classified as possessing PPWB traits engaged in more restorative behavior—regular exercise and at least eight hours of sleep per night—than those who did not. People with PPWB traits also had less sympathetic nervous system activation and greater parasympathetic control.

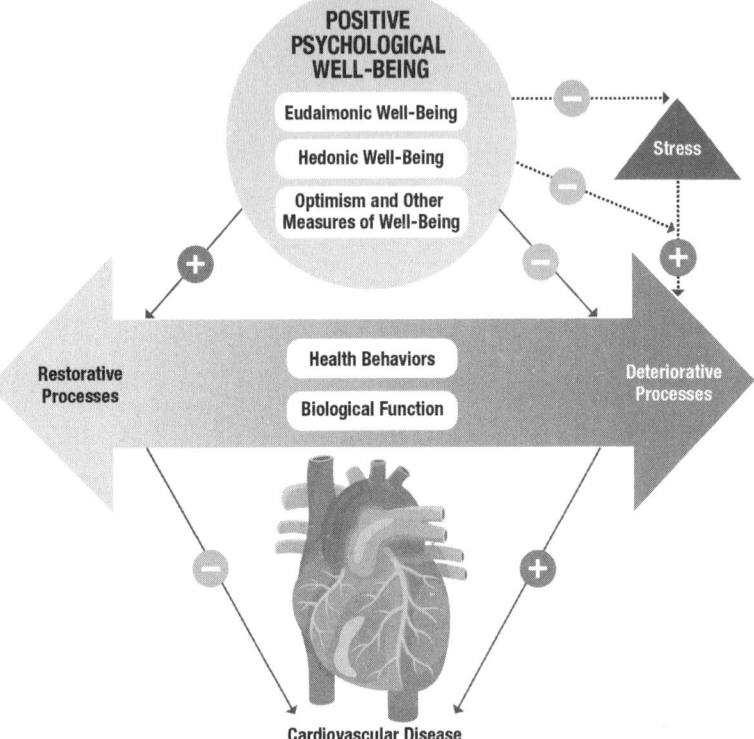

Fig. 3.4 The Relationship Between Well-Being and Cardiovascular Health

Let's revisit my patient, Kathy, by reviewing the information I just shared. What are her risk factors for heart disease? Genetically, she had a predisposition based on her parents' history of cardiovascular-related death. She had a history of anxiety and depression, which was treated in the past but was not currently being addressed, and she described herself as high-strung and Type A. My recommendations for Kathy included starting on a low dose of an antidepressant to help reduce her constant worry, exercising for thirty minutes per day, adopting a heart-healthy diet, practicing better sleep hygiene, and downloading a meditation app to teach her breathwork. In addition, I referred her to a cognitive behavioral therapist.

Fortunately, Kathy was feeling much better at her two-week follow-up appointment. She said, "Within a week, I started to feel the best I have felt in a long time." As a side benefit, her blood pressure readings had returned to normal.

What Are the Takeaways About Stress and Heart Disease?

- Emotional stress is an independent risk factor for heart disease.
- Women in menopause and patients with a preexisting history of psychiatric illness are at risk for some forms of stress-related heart disease.
- You can't change your genetic predisposition for heart disease, but you can change your behavior, which can reduce your risk.
- Learning to manage your parasympathetic nervous system can reduce the risk of many forms of stress-related heart disease.

CHAPTER 4

WHAT'S GOOD FOR THE HEART IS GOOD FOR THE BRAIN: THE LINK BETWEEN DEPRESSION AND HEART DISEASE

A good head and a good heart are always a formidable combination.
—NELSON MANDELA

In the 1930s, two long-term studies of depression found that depressed individuals had higher death rates from heart disease than those who did not, but this relationship was not truly appreciated until the 1980s. Since that time, studies of cardiovascular disease and depression have been conducted worldwide and consistently document the strong bidirectional relationship between the two disorders. In this chapter, I refer to all types of cardiovascular diseases as CVD.

Depression is the most common psychiatric illness, with a lifetime risk of 20 percent in the general population. Researchers project that, by 2030, depression will be one of the leading causes of disability worldwide. These two clinical conditions are intimately related, and a direct link between heart disease and depression exists in a bidirectional way. If this sounds familiar, that's because the theme of this book is that medical illness is not just in your head. Your brain and the rest of your major organs are interconnected, and what affects one affects all. If you suffer from CVD—heart disease, stroke, or hypertension—you are more likely to develop depression than someone without it. Conversely, if you have a diagnosis of depression, you are at a higher risk of developing cardiovascular disease compared to nondepressed individuals. In addition, people with more severe depression tend to experience more significant levels of cardiovascular disease, as well as increased rates of death. Research presented at the American College of Cardiology meeting in 2022 found that patients who develop depression after a cardiac diagnosis have an increased risk of death that is doubled if left untreated. In addition, untreated depression is a risk factor for a poor outcome after cardiovascular surgery. Although the prevalence of depression varies in patients with different types of coronary disease, approximately 15 percent of this population is affected. Depression doubles the risk of developing CVD, and the occurrence of depression in patients with acute myocardial infarction triples the mortality rate compared to those without depression.

How Does Unmanaged Depression Increase Your Risk of Heart Disease?

Current research indicates that the connection between depression and CVD is mediated through various channels. In this section, I review the roles of inflammation, stress hormones, lifestyle, and poor self-care as they relate to the onset or progression of cardiac disease. The good news is that each of these risk factors is subject to modification, which means there are ways to reduce your risk.

Inflammation: A Shared Pathway

A 2020 research review was conducted to understand the potential shared pathway of inflammation that impacts depression and cardiovascular disease. Stress is a significant risk factor for developing depression. In addition, stress causes our bodies to release more of the stress hormone cortisol. However, people who suffer from depression experience a persistence of stress and elevated levels of cortisol, which over time can cause wear and tear on the immune system, making it less effective. Eventually, immune cells become insensitive to the regulatory effects of cortisol and cause chronic inflammation and an increased susceptibility to diseases, including heart disease. Cortisol can cause your blood vessels to narrow, which means less blood flow to your vital organs and an elevation of your blood pressure, as discussed in the previous chapter. In addition, the ongoing constriction can cause damage to the lining of your blood vessels and lead to the buildup of plaques, a significant contributing factor to heart disease. Patients with depression also have stickier platelets, the component of blood responsible for clotting, which also contribute to the development of plaques.

A team at Cambridge University documented an association between high levels of a pro-inflammatory protein in the blood of children who later had an increased risk for the development of depression in young adulthood. Treatment with anti-inflammatory medications can lower the risk of cardiac-related death and may have implications for the treatment of depression as well. A recent large study from Boston's Brigham and Women's Hospital appears to confirm the hypothesis that inflammation plays a significant role in CVD. In this study, 10,061 patients with CVD from different populations in thirty-nine countries were randomized to receive injections of an anti-inflammation drug targeted explicitly for a pro-inflammatory protein. The medical status of these patients was followed for up to four years, and the results indicated significantly more favorable clinical outcomes for the patients who were given injections of the drug than for the control individuals who received a placebo. Recently, researchers have been investigating whether anti-inflammatory medications can be used successfully, either alone or in conjunction with traditional antidepressants, to improve outcomes in patients with depression. For example, nonsteroidal anti-inflammatory drugs (NSAIDs, such as celecoxib, naproxen, and ibuprofen) have been used in small research trials in patients with arthritis and depression. They reported a significant improvement in depressive symptoms that was unrelated to pain relief. One trial used statin drugs in combination with antidepressants for patients with moderate depression and found a decrease in depressive symptoms after six weeks. Statins are prescription medications prescribed to individuals who have elevated cholesterol and triglycerides. They work in the liver by inhibiting the process of creating cholesterol.

The shared mechanism involving inflammation is behind the comorbidity of CVD and depression, and is represented in the following diagram:

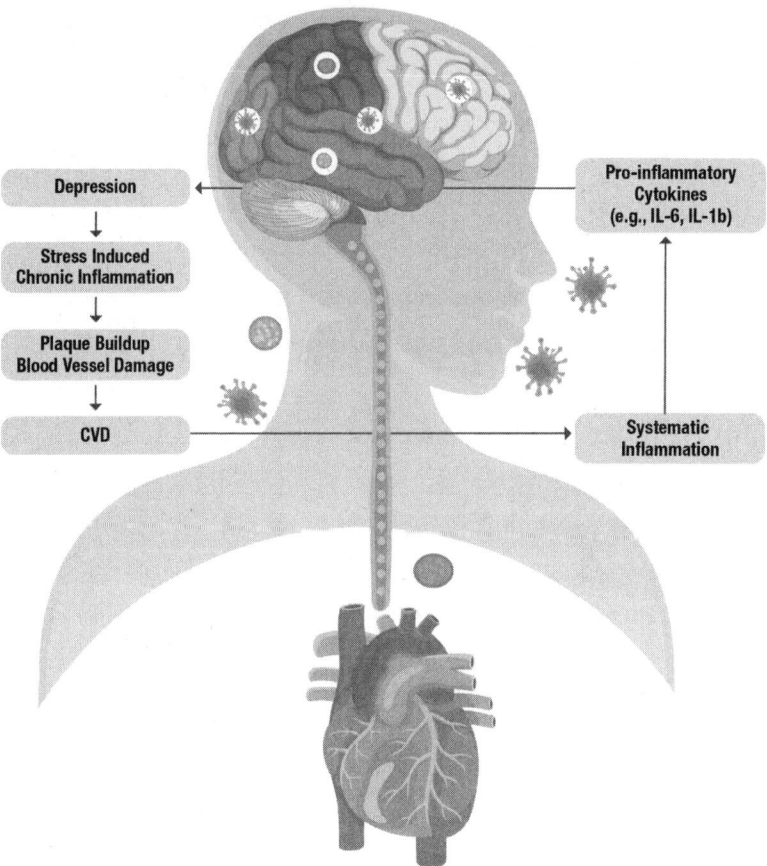

Fig. 4.1 Pathways for Depression and CVD

Understanding the shared mechanism can help investigators and practitioners develop strategies to lower the risk of each of these disorders. Some of the interventions showing success include nutritional interventions, practicing relaxation techniques, and treatment with anti-inflammatory medications.

- **Dietary interventions.** In later chapters, we discuss the effect of food on your mood and overall health. Research into the positive effects of an anti-inflammatory diet shows significant changes in decreasing your risk for heart disease and depression. Many foods and supplements—including omega-3, coenzyme Q10, turmeric, and even black pepper—help suppress the formation of one pro-inflammatory protein called IL-6. Another essential supplement that suppresses inflammation is vitamin D, which modulates your immune system by regulating cell signaling pathways through vitamin D receptors in your bones, muscles, kidneys, skin, and digestive tract. Vitamin D receptors have also been discovered in the central nervous system and play a role in your brain function. The receptors are particularly prevalent in an area of the brain involved in memory and emotion. Vitamin D deficiency can make it challenging for your body to manufacture the neurochemical serotonin, which is involved in numerous human behaviors and mental health disorders. One study reported that elderly patients who have coexisting cardiovascular disease and vitamin D deficiency reported higher rates of depression.
- **Stress management.** Some research studies report that using stress management strategies such as mind-body practices can lower your levels of some pro-inflammatory proteins. In a study comparing people who practice yoga daily versus those who do not, 41 percent of the practitioners were able to significantly reduce their levels of IL-6.

- **Anti-inflammatory drugs.** Colchicine is one of the oldest remedies still in use today. It is derived from a bulb known as autumn crocus. Its history as an herbal remedy for joint pain goes back to the 1500 BCE Egyptian manuscript the *Ebers Papyrus*. The active ingredient, colchicine, was isolated in the early 1800s and is used today as a purified natural product. Colchicine works by suppressing the components of inflammatory processes. In 2023, it was approved by the FDA under the name Lodoco as the first anti-inflammatory drug for cardiovascular disease.

Over nine thousand studies have investigated the role of the immune system in depression, particularly the role of inflammation. This is one of the theories that help to explain why patients with long COVID frequently describe symptoms of major depression. Low motivation is a symptom often seen in patients suffering from major depression. It is frequently described as a lack of drive or disinterest in starting or finishing tasks, especially those that are challenging or mundane. I can't even count all the times patients in my office say, "Isn't there just a pill for motivation?" And to that, I reply, "There isn't."

While there is no magic bullet or wonder drug that can push people to take action, a study published in *Nature* in 2024 reported the findings of research that looked at the effect of high levels of inflammation on the development of low motivation. The study enrolled forty-two subjects who were diagnosed with depression and also exhibited high levels of inflammation as measured by a blood test called C-reactive protein. They were randomly divided into two groups. One group of subjects received a single dose of an anti-inflammatory medication used to treat arthritis. The other group received a placebo. The researchers studied the subjects for two weeks, during which they were asked to perform various tasks and complete questionnaires designed to measure motivation levels. The results showed that the group that received the anti-inflammatory drug had an increased willingness to engage in tasks associated with rewards.

The Impact of Lifestyle and Poor Self-Care

In 2017, *Translational Psychiatry* published a fascinating article that described the genetic overlap between mood disorders and cardiovascular disease (CVD). The researchers cited the genetic contribution common to both mood disorders and CVD as being as high as 42 percent. Further, they suggested that the interactions between genetic factors and stress, physical exercise, diet, and lifestyle can influence the progression and severity of both disorders. The authors proposed that environmental factors could modulate the expression of genes involved in the pathways in our brain. Multiple studies further suggested that specific lifestyle factors were substantially involved in the association between depression and CVD risk. The journal *Nature* published the results of a study that investigated the impacts of gender and lifestyle on the association between depression and cardiovascular risk in a sample of British patients. In their population, those with high levels of depression who avoided nicotine, maintained a healthy weight, exercised regularly, and slept efficiently were able to lower their risk of cardiovascular disease, although this association was more pronounced in their female volunteers.

Depression is often associated with an unhealthy lifestyle, inactivity, smoking, alcohol abuse, obesity, and poor treatment adherence. Depression in those with heart failure decreases their ability to manage activities of daily living, such as physical exercise, good nutrition, and adherence to treatment, including medication. It can also contribute to social alienation. Lack of social support is an independent risk factor for CVD and is associated with a poor prognosis.

In general, when we talk about self-care, we refer to maintaining a healthy diet, sleeping adequately, engaging in activities that stimulate or give us pleasure, interacting with family or friends, moderating alcohol use, and avoiding habits that negatively affect our health, such as smoking. Major depression symptoms include altered sleep, appetite, energy, mood, or motivation, and decreased interest in usual activities. Poor self-care resulting from untreated depression has a significant impact on the development and maintenance of CVD.

If you are depressed, you may have little to no motivation to follow prescribed health guidelines, another way that depression and CVD are linked. Depression is a brain disorder, and when you are depressed, a part of your brain that is engaged in higher levels of functioning, called *executive functioning*, is not working up to speed.

In brain imaging studies, individuals who are depressed show low levels of activity in their prefrontal cortex. In addition, the severity of depression is often associated with the degree of decreased activity in this brain area. Because of the reduced activity, people who are depressed may show less motivation to practice self-care. We know, however, that making behavioral changes can improve your mood and, as a result, decrease your risk for cardiovascular disease. Such changes include the following:

- **Diet.** A healthy diet is essential for reducing your risk for heart disease. Depressed individuals sometimes suffer from a loss of appetite or engage in unhealthy eating habits, such as bingeing on sugar and fast foods. Diets high in salt and saturated fats are contributing factors to hypertension and increased buildup of plaques in the blood vessels, all contributing to the development of heart disease. In addition, poor dietary choices lead to obesity, which is an independent risk factor for heart disease.

- **Sleep.** Depressed individuals often report disturbed sleep, including difficulty falling asleep, frequent nighttime awakenings, waking up early, and being unable to return to sleep. This poorer quality of sleep contributes to decreased sleep time. It is essential to sleep adequately to keep your heart healthy. During sleep, your blood pressure decreases. If you have a sleep disturbance, your blood pressure stays higher for more extended periods and is a leading risk for heart disease and stroke. In addition, sleep deprivation contributes to overall body inflammation, which can elevate your risk of heart disease.
- **Energy.** Daytime fatigue is related to a decrease in physical activity. Let's face it: If you are tired, you are less likely to want to exercise. But exercise is a critical component of keeping your heart healthy. According to Johns Hopkins Medicine, exercise has many positive effects on heart health. These include lowering your blood pressure, keeping your weight in the healthy range, reducing overall inflammation, and strengthening your heart muscle.
- **Engaging in social activities.** If you are depressed, you may be less likely to engage in social activities with friends and family. Instead, you may choose to isolate, which is an unhealthy choice for your mood and your health. As

documented earlier in this chapter, low social support is correlated with a higher risk of CVD.

Takeaways for Lowering Your Risk of Depression and CVD

Depression is highly treatable. The *Journal of the American Heart Association* published its findings on psychiatric interventions in depressed patients with heart disease. They reviewed multiple large trials and found that selective serotonin reuptake inhibitors (SSRIs) are the most effective and safest medications to treat depression in those with heart disease. SSRIs, or selective serotonin reuptake inhibitors, are a class of antidepressant medications that increase the level of serotonin in the brain to improve mood. They work by blocking the reabsorption (reuptake) of serotonin, a chemical that helps regulate mood, sleep, and appetite Research trials using various SSRIs, including Prozac, Zoloft, and Lexapro, in patients with depression and heart disease reported that this class of antidepressant lowered self-reported depressive symptoms and improved cardiac outcomes in participants who were followed for up to one year. However, the results were different in patients with *heart failure*. For example, Dr. Christiane Angermann, a professor of cardiology at University Hospital Wurzburg, reported that the SSRI Lexapro was not helpful in treating hospitalized patients with heart failure and depression. She speculated, "Depression in heart failure may not be the same depression patients without heart failure get and who respond well to antidepressants. Heart failure is associated with biological changes that also cause depressive symptoms," she explained. "So it might be that an antidepressant is not the right drug to treat this depression." She further stated, "When we treat the heart failure very well, depression improves." Her theory is that greater degrees of heart failure in a patient will lead to a higher likelihood of an inflammatory process, which could be the cause of a poor antidepressant response. Although antidepressants may not be the best treatment for depression in patients with heart failure, she suggested that other approaches might be worth trying. When omega-3 fatty acids were prescribed either alone or in combination with antidepressants, the results were not improved.

Nonpharmacologic interventions like cognitive behavioral therapy were also reviewed. The researchers report more significant reductions in depressive symptoms with CBT therapy than other forms of psychotherapy. In a study at Washington University in St. Louis, researchers compared the results of CBT treatment of depression in heart failure patients with those who did not receive CBT but did receive the usual care (including education on heart failure by a cardiac nurse). Cognitive behavior therapy was effective compared to usual care for major depression in patients with heart failure. CBT did not improve self-care or physical functioning, but it did improve anxiety, fatigue, social functioning, and overall quality of life. An exploratory analysis suggested that the intervention might help to decrease the hospitalization rate in clinically depressed patients. The researchers concluded that major depression in heart failure may respond to CBT even if antidepressant therapy is unsuccessful.

MENDS Approach to Managing Mental Health and Heart Disease

Most medical illnesses are multifactorial in nature. My approach for managing these diagnoses is multifactorial as well, so I have created the MENDS approach. The abbreviation stands for medication, exercise, nutrition, dhyana, and sleep (social connections also).

Medication. Selective serotonin reuptake inhibitors are safe and effective for the treatment of depression and anxiety in patients with cardiovascular disease. Treatment with SSRIs may improve survival after myocardial infarction in patients with depression. Diagnosis and treatment of psychiatric morbidity should be incorporated into the clinical management of coronary heart disease and hypertension because, left untreated, they are independent risk factors for a worse outcome.

Exercise. Physical exercise is critical for improving mood and increasing parasympathetic activity in response to stress. Movement is a natural mood enhancer and helps maintain a healthy weight, lowers blood pressure, and decreases inflammation. Dr. Frank Doyle, a researcher at the Royal College of Surgeons in Dublin, published an article on the effect of exercise as a treatment option for patients with depression and heart disease. He concluded, "Exercise is likely to be the best treatment for depression following coronary artery disease. Our findings further highlight the clinical importance of exercise as a treatment as we see that it improves not only depression but also other important aspects of heart disease, such as lowering blood pressure and cholesterol, in these patients." Exercise can increase your sense of self-worth, self-confidence, sleep quality, and life satisfaction. Some studies document that people may seek social support during exercise interventions, which reduces loneliness.

Exercise can decrease inflammation, a risk factor for both depression and heart disease. In a twelve-week study of depressed elderly patients, aquatic exercise reduced depression and anxiety, as well as inflammation.

If the thought of jumping on a spin bike or going for a run is not your idea of a good time, especially if you feel depressed, many other activities can increase your heart rate. Gardening, washing your car, or cleaning your house can all be considered exercise. When you are running your errands, walk whenever possible. Park your car in the farthest space in the parking lot to get in some added steps. Take the stairs in your office instead of the elevator. Any physical activity that gets you off the couch can improve your mood. Even better, all your exercises do not have to be done in one session. Most experts recommend thirty minutes of vigorous exercise five times weekly for maximum benefit. You could split this into two fifteen-minute or even three ten-minute sessions daily. When it is broken down that way, it doesn't seem too overwhelming, does it?

Nutrition. Stress can deplete your body's stores of essential elements and vitamins. Recommended heart healthy diets include the Mediterranean diet or DASH. DASH stands for Dietary Approaches to Stop Hypertension, and it is an eating plan designed to help prevent or treat high blood pressure. The diet is rich in fruits, vegetables, whole grains, lean protein, and low-fat dairy, while being lower in sodium, saturated fats, and sugar. It can lower cholesterol, decrease your risk of developing plaques, lower your blood pressure, and maintain a balanced gut biome, improving brain function and mood.

Dhyana. Deep breathing is a great way to reduce the activation of your sympathetic nervous system, which controls your body's response to a perceived threat. Navy SEALs use a technique called "box breathing" to relax prior to engaging in a stressful procedure. It is called box breathing because it corresponds to four sides of a box:

BOX BREATHING

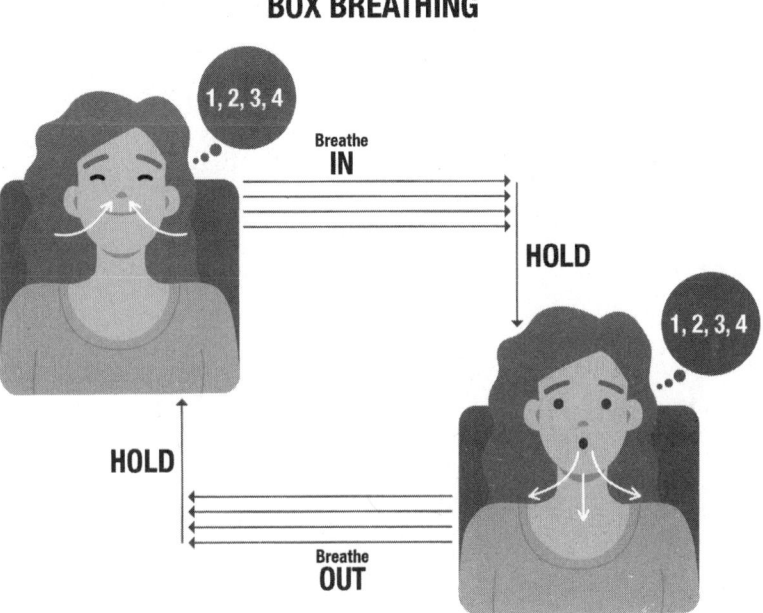

Fig. 4.2 Box Breathing

STEP 1: Breathe in, counting to four slowly. Feel the air enter your lungs.

STEP 2: Hold your breath for four seconds. Try to avoid inhaling or exhaling for four seconds.

STEP 3: Slowly exhale through your mouth for four seconds.

STEP 4: Wait for another four seconds before you breathe in again.

Repeat this exercise at least four times.

Sleep. In a study conducted in Canada in a community sample, investigators looked at the effect of sleep and depression on the development of heart disease. They found that higher levels of depression and disturbed sleep were independent risk factors for heart disease. In addition, the participants with both depression and a diagnosed sleep disorder in the two years prior to the study had an almost threefold increased risk of heart disease.

The American Heart Association recommends getting seven to nine hours of sleep per night. Sleeping later on the weekend does not make up for less sleep during the week. Researchers call this *sleep debt*. Try going to bed and waking up at the same time every day. Keep your room cool and dark. If you suspect you have sleep apnea, have it assessed. Treatment for sleep apnea lowers the risk of heart disease. Shut off your screens at least sixty minutes before you want to go to sleep, because focused activity and bright light activates your prefrontal cortex, the part of the brain you want to shut down in stages. Think of this as you would a computer: You don't just turn it off, you take several steps to shut it down appropriately.

What about a snoring bed partner? Sadly, I hear this all the time! Try wearing soft earplugs or using white noise (or another noise that may suit you, such as brown noise) to drown out the snores. In some cases, a couple may decide to sleep in separate rooms.

I'm adding another part of the S recommendation: **social connections.** Because low social support is correlated with depression and heart disease, spending time on social media sites can become stressful, not only because of what we might see there, but also because that time might be better spent visiting with friends, being outside, enjoying the weather, or reading a great book. Maintain your social connections; we humans are social beings. You need to have connections with people to feel supported. Finding a sense of community—whether at work, with a religious organization, or through shared activities, such as organized sports—is essential to your well-being. Enjoying a shared activity allows you to find support and foster relationships that can be supportive in difficult times, and it improves your overall health.

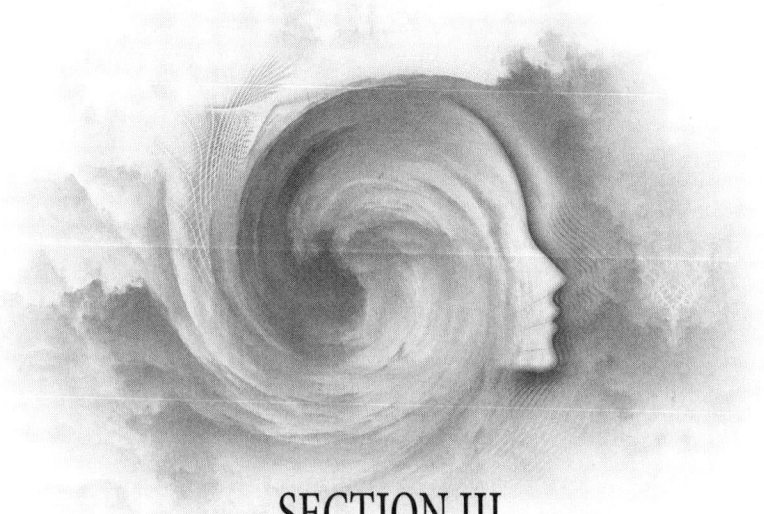

SECTION III

•••

YOUR TWO BRAINS

CHAPTER 5

BUTTERFLIES IN YOUR STOMACH AND OTHER GUT PHENOMENA

A person who belly laughs doesn't bellyache.
—SUSAN THURMAN

We are obsessed with our gut. Think about all the jargon that includes stomach or gut references: I hate his guts; that makes me sick to my stomach; I get butterflies in my stomach when I think of her; I have a gut feeling. We have a love-hate relationship with our gut, but one thing is for certain: We can't live without it. Our gut plays a vital role in our daily functioning. You certainly know about the gut's role in digestion and elimination, but did you know it also plays significant roles in immune function and mood modulation?

Remember how you felt in school on the day of an important test? What about getting behind the podium to present a lecture or entering your boss's office to ask for a raise? Some describe this as a "nervous stomach" or "feeling butterflies in their gut." These feelings are not imaginary. Your brain is linked directly to your digestive tract, and it began long ago when you were just a bundle of cells.

The Brain-Gut Connection

In simple terms, immature cells can develop into various types of organs and organ systems. Very early in an embryo's development, the process of *embryogenesis* grows a temporary structure called the *neural crest* that creates your brain and spinal cord. The same primitive structure provides the cells that develop into the enteric nervous system, also called the *second brain*. These cells reside in the wall of your gut. The direct connection between your brain and your gut is through a structure called the *vagus nerve*. Think of this as a major highway where traffic flows in two directions—from the brain to the gut and back to the brain. The traffic cops mediating the flow of information on this highway include your autonomic nervous system, sensory nerves, and hormones.

Understanding this connection explains the phenomenon of butterflies in your stomach. When you feel anxious, your brain sends a signal to the gut that says, "Time to worry." In a state of fight-or-flight, as discussed earlier, your sympathetic nervous system is in control. When your sympathetic nervous system is in charge, it slows digestion by directing blood away from your gut toward your large muscles. Remember, your body believes it is in survival mode, so it needs a way to evade danger. The reduced blood flow through your gut produces the characteristic feeling of something flitting around in the pit of your stomach. Your gut perceives this shortage of blood and oxygen, causing your sensory nerves to be unhappy with the situation. It may seem strange that your gut can influence your mood. However, in one study, scientists stimulated volunteers' vagus nerve at different electrical frequencies, which caused either a feeling of anxiety or well-being.

All That Pukes: Cyclic Vomiting Syndrome

Daniel was a thirty-year-old man who called for a consultation at the recommendation of a family friend. He'd attended Yale Law School and worked for a prestigious law firm in downtown Washington, DC. Although young, he had an impressive resume, having clerked for a US Court of Appeals judge before joining the firm as an associate, and he was well on his way to becoming a partner.

Daniel, who sported a mop of dirty blond hair that I could tell was carefully maintained with frequent blowouts and haircuts, arrived early for his appointment, wearing pressed khakis, a neat button-down shirt, his college tie, and shiny loafers. "I hope you can help me," he said. "I'm afraid this horrible situation will prevent me from getting where I want to go in my career."

Although Daniel had no difficulty completing his legal assignments, when asked to meet with clients or senior partners at a lunch or dinner engagement, he experienced an urgent need to vomit. His fear was so great that he would forgo eating for the entire day, reasoning that if his stomach was empty, he would not throw up. Unfortunately, despite this restriction, he often retched or experienced dry heaves. For Daniel, meetings with clients over meals were commonplace and unavoidable. Desperate, he turned to maladaptive ways to control his anxiety: consuming alcohol more frequently and smoking marijuana regularly to sleep.

Before our appointment, Daniel completed a full gastrointestinal workup. No medical reason for his symptoms could be found. He was otherwise healthy and had no family history of anxiety. What could have explained his symptoms, and what could I offer him?

The Role of Anxiety in Functional Gastrointestinal Disorders

Functional gastrointestinal disorders (FGID), such as irritable bowel syndrome (IBS), are diagnosed with specific symptoms (pain, gas, bloating, constipation, or diarrhea) *in the absence of objective findings on lab results or radiographic scans.* FGIDs are diagnosed in 35 to 70 percent of people at some point in their lives, more often in women.

After visiting many specialists who are unable to determine a physical cause for their complaints, patients who report these symptoms are often told, "It's all in your head," and referred to a psychiatrist. These patients tell me they feel misunderstood and dismissed by well-meaning but frustrated practitioners. Patients with FGID frequently have preexisting psychiatric disorders, most commonly anxiety and depression. In some studies, over 50 percent of patients with IBS had a coexisting psychiatric diagnosis. Researchers previously believed the psychiatric diagnosis led to the development of the gastrointestinal disease. However, they now recognize the reverse is true; in a significant proportion of individuals, the development of GI distress leads to psychiatric symptoms.

Daniel suffered from a FGID called *functional vomiting*, not a sexy-sounding diagnosis! Functional vomiting is defined as recurring, unexplained vomiting that occurs at least once per week and has no apparent medical cause. It is rare in the general population and has not received much investigation, but, as we've seen with Daniel, it can be very disabling.

In 2010, investigators in Beijing studied a group of patients with functional vomiting and found that the most common triggers for vomiting episodes were "emotional change and noxious stress." They concluded that the emotional triggers led to changes in physical sensations perceived by their gut, resulting in vomiting. Remember, the gut has a second brain; just like the brain in your head, it can perceive unpleasant physical sensations and respond with behavior to alleviate discomfort. Think of what happens when your brain perceives an itch: It makes you scratch.

In Daniel's case, the stress perceived by his gut led to the unwanted behavior. His history told the story of how this behavior began. Daniel felt "sick to his stomach" in grade school before taking a test. He attended a prestigious private all-boys school and was often bullied. His controlling mother micromanaged his course load and his sports activities. Daniel described a childhood in which he spent many weekends competing in sports at his mother's insistence. He would always throw up before a competitive tennis match, much preferring to be at home with his friends.

Daniel's father had a serious medical condition that affected him physically and mentally. Daniel told me he would get anxious at meals, watching his father struggle to feed himself. Dining out was particularly stressful since Daniel feared his father would trip and fall due to his poor balance, causing embarrassment to the family.

Significant stressors in his adult life included work pressure as he strove to make partner at the firm, the impending birth of his second child, and a decline in his father's health. After he and I discussed the likely connection between his anxiety and his physical symptoms, we arrived at a treatment plan. Daniel agreed to take an antidepressant. Although not clinically depressed, antidepressants can help treat anxiety disorders.

A 2011 study published in the *Journal of the Formosan Medical Association* reported successful treatment of functional vomiting in several patients using escitalopram (Lexapro), an SSRI. Ninety-five percent of your body's serotonin is found in your gut, where it acts as a signaling messenger. We think these medications work in the gut by acting as modulators. By treating the associated anxiety disorder, we can interrupt the messages coming from the brain to the gut that trigger the unwanted behavior. In addition to taking medication, Daniel started meditating, limited his alcohol intake, and stopped using marijuana. He agreed to see a cognitive behavioral therapist at some time in the future.

Nonpharmacologic strategies help treat FGID as well. In a 2020 *Journal of Ayurveda and Integrative Medicine* report, researchers conveyed their results after training fifty-four volunteers with FGID in Vaishvanara Agni meditation for fifty days. They asked the participants to complete a gastrointestinal quality-of-life questionnaire before and after training and found significant improvement in their gastrointestinal symptoms after completing the research trial. They concluded that the improvement was due to activation of the parasympathetic nervous system, which relaxes the body and improves digestion.

A Badass and Her Bad Ass

Angela was a former New Yorker of Italian heritage with bright red hair and nails to match. She was a lively seventy-year-old woman whose speech was sprinkled with humor, and she used dramatic hand gestures to emphasize her points. Before retirement, she and her husband were professors at a local university. Angela's area of expertise was art history. Her daughter, who was a patient of mine, referred her to me for assistance in managing her FGID.

"So, this problem started forty years ago, and it's a pain in my ass!" Angela said.

I must admit, I was very drawn in by her forthright manner.

"You don't mind if I curse, do you, Doc?" she asked.

"No, go right ahead. Feel free to explain things in whatever way works best for you," I told her.

Angela continued, "The panic attacks started when I was in the first trimester of my first pregnancy. I started having pains right here." She pointed to the center of her abdomen. "It hurt like hell, and I had to go poop multiple times a day. It's like my body was trying to tell me something was wrong, and sure enough something did go very wrong."

Angela started tearing up, and I pointed to the box of tissues on my table, encouraging her to take some. Angela's pregnancy did not end well. The baby was premature and died shortly after birth.

"God didn't want me to have that baby, but it was just so very hard. Robert [her husband] and I held her, that sweet, small, precious baby, and then she just stopped breathing." Angela was crying openly at this deeply painful memory.

"Why don't you take a moment and catch your breath?" I suggested.

Angela continued sobbing, blew her nose, and said she was ready to continue. "It was so hard to lose her, but it was so long ago. One good thing that came out of that was that I have two grown daughters and three grandchildren. If the first one had lived, I wouldn't have the family I now have. Robert and I married when we were older, in our thirties, which I know is common now, but it wasn't when we were young. It took awhile for me to conceive again, and we needed infertility help."

Angela started crying again. "A week after Libby was born, my parents were visiting their friends. They were supposed to come see us and the baby the following weekend. On their way home from dinner, they were hit by a drunk driver and died at the scene of the accident. That was a long time ago, but the problem with my guts and always having to go worsened after that. I remember my father had problems with his stomach. My mother used to call him 'weak guts' because he would develop diarrhea anytime things became stressful. The roof needed repair; Dad was in the toilet. The stock market was off, and so was Dad—off to the bathroom, that is!"

Both of her daughters suffered from anxiety disorders, but neither had been diagnosed with a functional gastrointestinal disorder.

Because of her condition, Angela engaged in a detailed ritual to travel even short distances from her home. She said, "If I want to go see my daughter in North Carolina, I must starve myself for almost forty-eight hours so my gut will be empty, and I won't have to use the bathroom. My biggest fear is if I must go and I'm in a confined space with no way out."

Angela loved visiting museums, especially art museums downtown, but rarely did so because it meant a trip on the Metro in a confined space with no bathroom.

"Since I now live such a controlled and limited life, the panic attacks have decreased. But I miss my old life and want to be able to see friends and enjoy the city since I'm retired. It's so hard since I always have to think ahead and make a contingency plan because the pain can just come on so unpredictably. I need you to help me develop a strategy for dealing with this. I don't want to spend the rest of my life at the mercy of my ass!"

I Don't Have Irritable Bowel, I Have Vindictive Bowel!

Frances was referred to me by her gastroenterologist to help manage her irritable bowel syndrome. A petite woman in her early sixties, she arrived at my office perfectly put together. Her colored, dirty-blond hair was meticulously coifed. Her matching cream-colored sweater, slacks, and shoes offered a beautiful monochromatic look worthy of a catalog cover. Her makeup was flawless, natural, and just the right touch. I was impressed, maybe even a bit envious. I never look that put together! As I've come to know, outward appearances never tell the full story or the pain someone is experiencing.

"I feel like it controls me," Frances said as she sat across from me on my couch.

"Tell me more," I responded as I picked up my pad and pen, ready to document her history.

"My symptoms started when my mother was diagnosed with breast cancer, which was just before my first daughter was born. I would get these awful stomach pains that came on out of nowhere. If I didn't get to the bathroom quickly, I could easily soil myself, which happened more than once, and was so incredibly embarrassing.

"I was so overwhelmed taking care of my mother, and then I gave birth to my child, which was exhausting. I wasn't sleeping, I hardly ate, and I was just so anxious all the time."

"Did you have a history of being anxious before these events took place?" I inquired.

"My childhood was tough," she said. "I grew up outside Philly, the eldest girl in a family of four children. My father was mostly absent. He worked all the time, and when he was home, all he wanted to do was sit in front of the TV, read the paper, and drink beer. My mother was very difficult. She probably had lifelong depression, which was never treated, so she would have these rages when she would yell, throw things, and be so critical. It didn't matter what I did, whatever it was, she told me it was wrong. I was expected to be her servant and wait on her hand and foot. I had to miss school to take care of her when she was pregnant with my brother."

"Did you ever tell anyone, like a teacher or relative, about what was happening?" I asked.

"I was a shy kid, not a fighter like my younger sister. I just wanted to keep the peace so she wouldn't get angry, so I did what I thought would make that happen. It didn't matter, though. Even if I cleaned the house, did the laundry, and helped to cook dinner, she constantly criticized.

"I was fifteen when my baby brother was born. When I came home from school, I would feed him. My mother was very manipulative. She would threaten suicide frequently and made several overdose attempts, which led to her hospitalizations. Of course, when she was away, I was expected to take over the household duties for her."

"Francis, that sounds like the kind of childhood that could make anyone anxious. Was there anyone you could turn to for support?" I was scribbling notes but looked up to see her expression.

"Not really. My mother's brother was funny. I liked him, but he had an edge to him, too. We used to go to the New Jersey beaches for vacations in the summer. One time, he almost drowned me while we were playing in the water. Another time, he stepped on my foot on purpose so I would cry. I told my mother, but she said, 'Don't make any trouble.'"

"If I had seen you then, I would have told you that you needed a parent-ectomy—meaning you had to get away from your environment," I said.

Frances laughed at that. "It got better when I married my husband and left home." Frances was twenty at the time.

Unfortunately, Frances later suffered the loss of her mother and then her younger sister, to whom she was very close. Her IBS symptoms grew worse during those times. She had conflicted feelings about her mother but deeply loved her sister, and that was what really tipped the scales.

She was so private and embarrassed by her symptoms that she did her best to hide them from her children. When they asked, "What's wrong, Mama?" after her extended periods in the bathroom, she would answer, "Oh, it's nothing. Mama just ate something that made her tummy ache."

A full gastrointestinal workup failed to reveal a cause for her symptoms. Francis said her IBS controlled her behavior and limited her activity. Although she did not restrict food, she had limited her activity outside her home because her symptoms of severe pain and diarrhea could occur at any time and last for up to three hours.

Frances considered herself a social person who liked to be with friends. However, she and her husband, Jack, had limited their social activities because she feared embarrassing herself by spending hours in the bathroom.

"One really bad incident happened when I was on my way to attend a close friend's family celebration. We had talked about this for months, and she and I were really looking forward to reuniting again. Jack and I were on our way, on the New Jersey Turnpike, when it happened. I had severe stomach pain, and I knew the diarrhea wouldn't be far behind. I told Jack, 'We must stop. I need to go!' We were still several miles from a rest stop, so we had to take a detour to find me a bathroom pronto.

"When we got there, I ran out of the car and into the restroom. This episode was bad; it went on for like three hours. I knew we were going to miss the affair, and I was mortified that I would have to explain this to my friend."

"So, what happened?"

"I didn't call her for a few days. I was too scared to. When I finally did, she was so nice, but I didn't tell her the truth. I said the car broke down and my cell phone had died, so I couldn't reach her."

Psychological disorders like anxiety play an important role in individuals who suffer from functional gastrointestinal disorders. Studies report that up to 50 percent of all patients with IBS have a psychiatric diagnosis. Both Frances and Angela, who you met earlier, experienced the onset of gastrointestinal disorders during times of extreme stress. Interestingly, both noted that their symptoms began either during or after a pregnancy and worsened around the time a loved one died. The idea that stress can exacerbate many medical illnesses is generally well accepted. However, the mechanism for how this occurs has not yet been scientifically defined.

Early Trauma and Functional Gastrointestinal Disorders

IBS is a common disorder experienced by 10 to 15 percent of the general adult population. Because of the large number of people afflicted with IBS, it has adversely impacted healthcare costs and even the American economy. The high prevalence of illness due to IBS accounts for an estimated $1.7 billion in annual direct medical costs in the United States and an estimated $20 billion in indirect costs due to worker absenteeism.

Evidence from longitudinal studies—those that follow subjects from childhood to adulthood—suggests that adults with IBS experienced recurrent functional abdominal pain and constipation as children. For example, an article published in the *American Journal of Gastroenterology* reported that in their study group, individuals who reported IBS in their late twenties were more likely to have reported histories of abdominal pain and constipation as children than age-matched healthy subjects. In addition, patients with IBS differed from nonpatients because they reported more frequent visits to doctors as children with symptoms of abdominal discomfort but also more headaches and worse overall health.

Several research studies have identified trauma-related risk factors during infancy that may lead to IBS symptoms in adults. One study looked at early intrauterine growth delay as a predisposing risk factor. Researchers in Norway followed twelve thousand sets of twins over a two-year period. They found that the twins with low birth weights were significantly more likely to develop IBS in later years, and the symptoms tended to be more severe.

A different study looked at trauma during birth as a risk factor for the later development of IBS. Babies who required gastric suctioning at birth were more likely to need treatment for IBS later in life.

Frances had a long and contentious relationship with a mentally ill mother that continued until her mother's death. Angela lived in a home with a chronically ill father who repeatedly complained of gastrointestinal symptoms. Multiple researchers have reported that adults with IBS were more likely to have experienced physical, verbal, or sexual abuse as children. Parental deprivation during childhood was also reported as a significant risk factor. In one research study, over 60 percent of participants with IBS reported unsatisfactory relationships with at least one parent, or losing a parent due to death, separation, or divorce.

Researchers hypothesize that prenatal, early infancy, and childhood traumatic events may sensitize an individual to the presence of functional gastrointestinal symptoms later in life. Other investigators suggest that injurious childhood events, or possibly prenatal trauma, can overly stimulate the sensory system in the gut itself so that affected individuals are overly vigilant about any perceived alteration in gut activity.

Like Parent, Like Child? How Modeling of Illness Behavior Is Linked to IBS

Individuals with IBS may develop illness behavior as a result of exposure to their parents' reactions to their own symptoms. Both Angela and Frances grew up in families where at least one parent exhibited the "sick role." Social learning of illness behavior can occur in several ways. When parents respond to their child's abdominal complaints with excessive attention, this behavior is reinforced. What child doesn't want more attention?

When parents with IBS behave in a way that demonstrates a preoccupation with illness, this may reinforce sick behavior as being positive so that it will occur with increased frequency in their children. In support of this theory, one researcher found that individuals with IBS and illness behavior were more likely to report childhood reinforcement of illness behavior as they recalled being given gifts or special foods when they had an illness.

An interesting study looked at the possible effect of birth order and number of siblings in the family of adults suffering from FGID. Individuals with unexplained abdominal pain reported an average of 5.4 siblings versus an average of four siblings in the group that had verifiable abdominal pain. The authors theorized that individuals in larger families tended to report symptoms in order to gain attention.

Stress Messes with Your Gut Biome

Psychological stress significantly influences your gut biome. In an interesting study using college students as volunteers, a group of researchers reported that students had less healthy bacteria in their fecal matter during exam times than at other times during the school year. Other researchers reported a lack of immune-supporting bacteria in patients who are clinically depressed. Although we know psychological stress is associated with an altered gut environment, the cause-and-effect relationship has not been effectively established. Despite this, researchers postulate several plausible mechanisms to explain this phenomenon:

- **The junk food theory.** Exposure to stress can trigger comfort eating, which includes ultra-processed foods high in sugar, fat, and salt. These types of foods can lead to alterations in the gut environment.
- **The Swiss cheese theory.** Chronic stress may lead to a decrease in motility or movement through the digestive tract and a decrease in protective intestinal mucus. Imagine this as you would a piece of Swiss cheese. The more holes, the more destructive elements can pass through. This impacts digestion, absorption, and elimination, and may ultimately cause

an overgrowth of pathological or unwanted bacteria at the expense of your necessary healthy bacteria.

According to an article in *World Journal of Gastroenterology*, stress-induced changes in the gut environment may play a key role in how a person develops IBS.

Manage the Stress, Manage the FGID Symptoms

Now that we have reviewed the meaning of FGID and its possible causes, and explored its connection to stress, this section provides you with some practical tools to manage your symptoms.

Antidepressants have effects that go beyond stabilizing a person's mood. They can affect many aspects of the body, especially the digestive system. It is becoming common for these drugs to be called *neuromodulators* rather than antidepressants because they widely target the nervous system. For individuals with IBS, they have a positive impact on gut motility—contractions of the digestive tract that move nutrients through the gut and help with absorption and elimination. They may also diminish the gut's sensitivity to pain, which is called *visceral sensitivity*. Most of the patients I see in my practice who have GI disorders also suffer from some form of anxiety. For those who have anxiety as well as FGID, treating the underlying anxiety may reduce the incidence of IBS episodes.

Angela agreed to take a low dose of an antidepressant called Zoloft. This medication specifically targets a neurotransmitter called serotonin. Surprising fact: There are more serotonin receptors in your gut than in your brain. Receptors are the landing sites for brain chemicals or neurotransmitters. Think of this as a lock and key. The key is the antidepressant; the lock is the receptor. The appropriate key must fit for the lock to work. SSRIs work because they slow the breakdown and reabsorption of serotonin into the spaces between nerve cells.

It took a little while, but with time and patience, I was able to raise Angela's dose from one that is used in a pediatric population to one that is therapeutic to treat her anxiety and abdominal pain. Slowly, she started going out again and even began to use the Metro. I haven't seen her in a few years, which I hope is good news. The last time we met, she was doing well and was grateful.

"Doc, you did it! I just returned from visiting my daughter in North Carolina, and I didn't have to starve myself before getting in the car. We just planned the route so that if I had to go, we would stop at rest stops every hour or so. Knowing I could do that, and taking the meds, made the trip possible."

As I like to remind my patients, medication isn't the answer for everyone. It is a tool, much like glasses, which help you see better but do not improve your eyesight. In addition to medication, or for those who choose not to take medicine, I also encourage the following protocols.

Calm Your Brain, Calm Your Gut: Cognitive Behavioral Therapy

CBT is a research-based, active therapeutic approach. In CBT, the therapist and patient work as a team to set treatment goals, assign homework, evaluate the effectiveness of techniques, and determine when to stop treatment. CBT targets problem areas using specific cognitive and behavioral techniques. A significant body of research indicates that CBT is effective in reducing IBS symptoms of abdominal pain, diarrhea, and constipation.

Cognitive behavioral therapy for IBS usually involves teaching the individual specific strategies for calming the body, coping with unpleasant symptoms, and learning to face difficult situations. Any or all of the above techniques might be used, depending on the needs of the individual. In general, symptom improvement seen following a course of CBT can be expected to continue after treatment has ended. In its 2020 research review, the *American College of Gastroenterology* recommends CBT as a viable treatment for IBS.

Daniel, the attorney we met earlier, chose Zoloft, but for months, he continued to have bouts of dry heaves in the morning before going to work. I encouraged him to see a cognitive behavioral therapist I know. With the addition of this mode of therapy, his vomiting has essentially gone into remission. A follow-up with Daniel six months later was a pleasant surprise. He told me he no longer drinks or uses marijuana, he walks every day, but best of all, he quit his job! Daniel realized his job was a significant source of stress, but after reviewing his investment portfolio, he decided he could afford to take a less lucrative but lower-stress job in the public sector. He told me he was much happier, and he even looked more relaxed.

I see Frances every few years, often after a significant stressor leads to a recurrence of her IBS symptoms. My initial treatment with Celexa, another selective serotonin reuptake inhibitor, worked beautifully for several months. However, her older daughter began having marital issues, and Francis experienced stress as a result. Unfortunately, the gastrointestinal symptoms returned. She agreed to a twelve-week course of CBT, which was mostly successful, except she did not always complete the homework the therapist prescribed. She relapsed again, and this time, in addition to medication and CBT, I suggested regular exercise.

Mobility leads to motility: Exercise works wonders for the brain and body. Remember, IBS and other FGID disorders are disorders of the brain-gut interaction. According to Dr. Brennan Spiegel, a gastroenterologist, professor of medicine and public health, and the director of Health Services Research at Cedars-Sinai in Los Angeles, "Exercise is part of the behavioral health and holistic care necessary to improve the brain-gut axis and outcomes in IBS." You do not have to be a marathon runner to benefit from exercise. Getting in your daily steps with a walk or a light jog burns calories, helps regulate blood sugar levels, and works several large muscle groups. A study published in May 2020 in *PLOS One* found that the more steps people with IBS took per day, the less severe their symptoms. In a study published in February 2018 in the *Journal of Bodywork and Movement Therapies*, participants who did six weeks of exercise on a treadmill for just thirty minutes three times a week saw significant improvement in their IBS symptoms and their mood.

Hopping on a bike, whether stationary or on the road, is an excellent workout for your legs and heart. A study published in January 2015 in the *World Journal of Gastroenterology* found that IBS patients who maintained a cycling or other exercise habit had improved symptoms and overall health if they continued with this strategy—even five years after they started exercising.

Frances and her husband created a home gym in their basement. They exercise regularly, have each lost fifteen pounds, and so far, her IBS is in remission. Although it is possible her symptoms will return, she now has some tools in her psychological toolbox to manage them.

In addition to exercise, here are some other strategies to try.

Stretch and Relax: Your Gut Will Love You for It

Yoga improves mood and digestion. A review published in December 2019 in *Digestive Diseases and Sciences* found that study participants who started a yoga practice improved their digestion, reduced their IBS symptoms, and felt stronger. They also reported less depression and anxiety.

Mindfulness Meditation

Bruce Naliboff, PhD, a clinical professor in the department of psychiatry and biobehavioral sciences at UCLA's David Geffen School of Medicine, led a team of researchers who followed sixty-eight IBS patients through an eight-week mindfulness-based stress reduction class that included weekly group trainings and daily thirty-minute meditation sessions at home. More than 70 percent of participants in the study reported a reduction in the severity of their IBS symptoms following the training, and benefits continued three months after its conclusion. Additionally, participants reported significant improvements in their quality of life and reductions in anxiety associated with their IBS symptoms.

Key Connections

- Your gut and brain are intimately connected. They are born of the same cloth and continue their close communication throughout our lives. They are best friends who share their ups and downs constantly. They like to share their feelings, so if one is anxious, the other picks up the vibe and is worried. In addition to sharing stress and anxiety, they communicate about diet (just like friends do!). Healthy eating will improve your gut environment and help your brain feel less stressed.

- There are many ways to reduce stress in your life and, by extension, reduce stress levels in your gut and brain. So get out there and try some of these strategies. Be kind to yourself. You do not have to make all these changes at once, and you can even just do some of them. Making a single change will likely lead to some improvement in your health and may make you more motivated to try other suggestions. Remember, it's progress, not perfection!

This chapter introduced the idea of stress as a prominent contributor to the development of FGID. In the next chapter, we see how another common psychiatric disorder, depression, plays a role in many gastrointestinal diseases and how the reverse may also be true. If your gut is depressed, it can make your brain experience the same symptoms.

CHAPTER 6

IS YOUR STOMACH DEPRESSED? THE LINK BETWEEN YOUR GUT AND MOOD

All disease begins in the gut.
—HIPPOCRATES

In the previous chapter, I discussed the development of the gut-brain connection and how these two act like besties, always sending signals to each other. In this chapter, I describe what we know about how your gut environment (also known as the biome) is involved in mood disorders.

The vast community of bacteria, viruses, fungi, and other microorganisms (microbes) living in our intestines plays a crucial role in regulating our physical and mental health. Although many microbes make up our gut environment, bacteria are the most frequently studied. The entire collection of microorganisms is referred to as the *gut biome*. You may be surprised that the human body contains more bacterial cells than human cells! Each group of microorganisms plays a different role in our body. Many support our health, but some can cause disease.

The first time we are exposed to microbes is as infants during the passage through our mother's birth canal. However, some newer research shows that developing fetuses can come into contact with some of their mother's microbes while still developing in the womb. An infant's intestines have little microbial diversity. However, as the baby grows and starts consuming either breast milk or formula, the population of microbes expands. Interestingly, the baby's fetal environment also plays a role. For example, Dr. William Turpin's 2022 study showed that babies whose mothers owned pets during their pregnancy had a much more varied gut biome than those who did not.

Think of your gut biome as a garden where some of the inhabitants benefit the growth and welfare of the garden (good microbes) and some are potentially toxic. Just like a good garden is composed of a diverse group of plants, your body and overall health are better when a diverse group of microorganisms populate your gut. Generally, these diverse species live in harmony within our intestines. Sometimes, however, environmental changes, trauma, illness, and even prescribed medications can lead to an imbalance called *dysbiosis*. When this happens, it can contribute to various kinds of disease, including psychiatric illness.

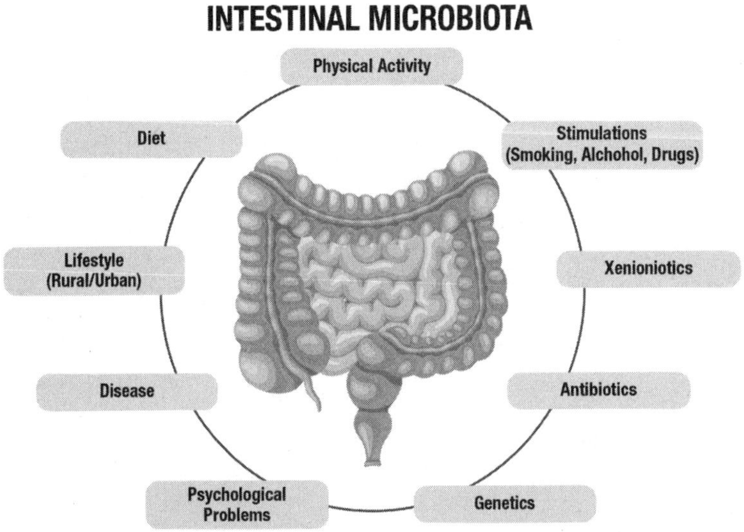

INTESTINAL MICROBIOTA

- Physical Activity
- Diet
- Stimulations (Smoking, Alchohol, Drugs)
- Lifestyle (Rural/Urban)
- Xenioniotics
- Disease
- Antibiotics
- Psychological Problems
- Genetics

Fig. 6.1 Multiple Variables Influence the Gut Environment

What Happens When Dysbiosis Occurs?

The blood-brain barrier (BBB) is a crucial central nervous system immune component. It is made up of many cell types and acts as a roadblock to bacteria, fungi, viruses, or parasites that may be circulating in your bloodstream. Similarly, the cells that line your intestines form a membrane that protects your gut from circulating invaders and prevents toxic elements of your biome from entering your bloodstream. Some of these cells are connected by structures called *tight junctions*. This arrangement ensures that only the smallest particles can pass between cells. Figure 6.2 depicts a healthy gut membrane on the left with tight junctions compared with a damaged membrane on the right with spaces between cells.

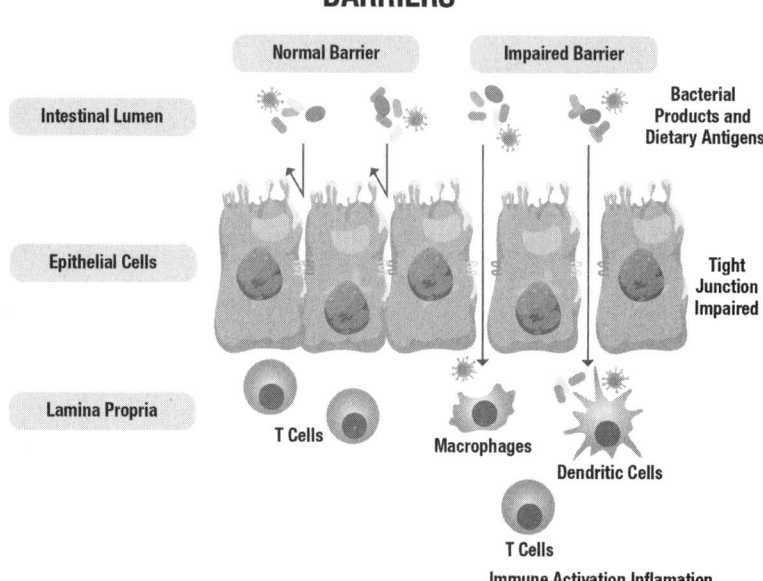

Fig. 6.2. Comparison Between a Healthy Versus Damaged Gut Membrane

Once this occurs, bacterial products and dietary toxins can enter and activate your immune system. Your gut is not only involved in digesting and elimination—it is also a significant part of your immune system.

What Is Leaky Gut?

Leaky gut occurs when toxic elements travel across your gut wall. Scientists call it *increased intestinal permeability* or *intestinal hyperpermeability*. A small amount of leakiness is normal. These minor leaks remind your immune system not to overreact to foods and normal gut bacteria. But an increase in leakiness could harm your health. For example, if your small intestine wall is compromised, you may absorb undigested food, toxins, and bacteria.

Leaky gut syndrome, long associated with celiac disease (CD), has attracted a good deal of attention in recent years. As you age, and under specific conditions, small components of your gut's bacterial metabolism can leak out and travel to distant sites in your body. If one of the distant sites is the brain, these toxic elements can pass the BBB and reach the central nervous system. Celiac disease is a genetic autoimmune condition. A similar condition, gluten sensitivity, does not appear to be genetic or autoimmune, and gluten intolerance has been linked to mood disorders. In humans, symptoms associated with CD are not limited to the GI tract. We also see associated skin, neurologic, and psychiatric disorders. Depression is twice as common in patients with celiac disease than in those without the disorder. The relationship of celiac disease to neurologic and psychiatric complications has been observed for over forty years. However, a significant proportion of people with CD do not have GI symptoms as their prime complaint. Neurologic and psychiatric complications seen in gluten-sensitive patients may be the first symptoms to arise in some patients suffering from this disease.

Bread, Brains, and the Blues: What Is the Possible Link?

- Various studies have suggested a possible link between brain functions and malabsorption, the inability to properly absorb nutrients from food.
- When the intestines are damaged, more toxic substances can pass through the gut and into the bloodstream, and some of these substances impact brain function.
- Adopting a gluten-free diet can help alleviate symptoms of depression for some people with CD.
- Depression can occur in some people after their diagnosis as well, because of the significant impact on their daily life,

and the challenges and stress that can come with managing a chronic condition, as well as a restrictive diet.
- Depression has also been linked to nonceliac gluten sensitivity.

Despite the somewhat conflicting results regarding which psychological disorders are associated with celiac disease, researchers generally agree that depression and anxiety are the most commonly reported. The prevalence of depression in celiac disease varies between 6 percent and 57 percent, with the lowest rate occurring among people who follow a gluten-free diet. Despite improvements in GI symptoms when following this diet, some patients continue to report depressive symptoms. Some researchers have speculated that having such a restrictive diet could be enough to trigger a sense of hopelessness in some patients, but it turns out to be much more complicated. For example, scientists report that some patients with CD have lower levels of tryptophan (a building block of one of our neurotransmitters, serotonin) and vitamin B, and less blood flow to the brain. Celiac disease is a chronic disease, and since lifelong adherence to a gluten-free diet is demanding and costly, the psychological aspects for these patients are significant.

What Can You Do If You Suffer from Celiac Disease and Depression?

Lifelong elimination of gluten from your diet is still the first-line treatment for celiac disease. In some studies, eliminating gluten led to improvement in depressive symptoms within weeks. However, for some people, even strict elimination of gluten does not alleviate depression. The proportion of people still depressed after adhering to a strict diet was thought to be due to malnutrition, which results from the elimination of necessary nutrients or vitamins found in gluten products.

There's good news on the nutritional front. Although recovery from celiac disease-related disorders requires strict adherence to a gluten-free diet, grocery shelves are full of gluten-free foods and products, and many restaurants now offer gluten-free alternatives on their menus.

The Celiac Disease Foundation lists gluten-free menus and restaurants that offer gluten-free dining (https://celiac.org/). Please visit the References section at the end of this book for more details.

Even in people who do not suffer from gluten sensitivity or CD, gut dysbiosis is associated with the progression or worsening of mood disorders. In the previous chapter, I mentioned that researchers used to think that anxiety and depression caused functional bowel problems. However, we have learned that the reverse is probably true. Since the mid-2010s, the potential role of the gut environment in the development of mood disorders has led to increased research in this area.

Evidence Linking Gut Microbiome and Mood Disorders

Both human and animal studies provide increasing evidence suggesting a strong link between gut biome composition and development of psychological disorders, such as depression and anxiety. For example,

- Animal studies showed that exposure to antibiotics or intestinal toxins led to a distinct change in their behavior, which implied an impact on their brains when their intestinal bacterial status changed.

- Animals whose gut microbiome is altered negatively show reduced brain-derived neurotrophic factor (BDNF) levels and decreased sensitization of their serotonin receptors. The animals whose microbiome was altered in a negative way had lower levels of a protein that promotes the growth and survival of new neurons. In addition, their brain receptors were made less sensitive to serotonin.
- In humans, BDNF plays a pivotal role in the brain and the central nervous system. It helps nerve cells grow, develop, and survive. In addition, it helps regulate neuroplasticity, the ability of aspects of your nervous system to change and adapt over time. Some of its other functions include helping to form long-term memory, impacting your mood, sleep patterns, and eating patterns. In short, it is a big deal! Over the past decade, researchers have been looking at the emerging role of gut microorganisms as a contributor to nerve formation and BDNF production. Studies have already shown that reduced BDNF levels can lead to the development of mood disorders.
- Patients diagnosed with major depressive disorder (MDD) have a different fecal microbiome composition compared to healthy volunteers. Several studies have found that people with depression often have distinct gut microbiota compared to healthy individuals. For example, people with depression may have reduced microbial diversity and lower levels of beneficial bacteria like *Bifidobacteria* and *Lactobacilli*. Conversely, those with a more balanced gut microbiome have better mental health outcomes.

Believe it or not, microorganisms can emit neurotransmitters, the chemical messengers that carry signals between nerve cells, muscles, and glands. Many of these neurotransmitters are involved in regulating memory, attention, and mood. Since 90 percent of your body's serotonin resides in your gut, and serotonin is highly influential in many brain functions such as sleep, mood, and appetite, any dysregulation in the composition of the gut microorganisms can cause changes in any or all of these functions.

Some Antidepressants Have Antimicrobial Effects

An older antidepressant class called MAO inhibitors is not often used today. These drugs are more cumbersome because patients must be cautious about diet and medication interactions. However, early research on this class of drugs showed that they have antibiotic activity and can effectively treat some infectious diseases. Another group of older antidepressants, tricyclics, showed antibacterial effects against bacteria such as *E. coli* in laboratory studies.

Most practitioners use the more common antidepressants, such as SSRIs, to treat mood disorders. Since they are dosed only once a day, many patients find them more convenient to take, and they have fewer side effects. In addition, a fascinating secondary effect of using SSRIs also showed promise in decreasing inflammatory properties. Blocking reuptake makes more serotonin available to help pass messages between brain cells. SSRIs are called *selective* because they mainly affect serotonin.

However, they also have antibiotic activity against some bacteria, although the precise mechanism is poorly understood. During the COVID-19 pandemic, a research group from Stanford and the University of California, San Francisco, published their work, which analyzed electronic health records from an extensive database that had information from almost 500,000 patients across the United

States. This included 83,584 adult patients diagnosed with COVID between January and September 2020. Of those, 3,401 patients were prescribed two SSRIs, fluoxetine and fluvoxamine. The results showed that patients taking fluoxetine were 28 percent less likely to die; those taking either fluoxetine or fluvoxamine were 26 percent less likely to die, and the entire group of patients taking any SSRI was 8 percent less likely to die than the matched patient controls. Why were these SSRIs effective in treating COVID? They work by increasing the brain's level of serotonin, which aside from improving mood and decreasing anxiety, also influences the immune system. In patients with COVID, they may prevent or limit the cytokine release process that is partly responsible for worsening the inflammatory component of the illness.

Fecal Transplants Can Improve Symptoms of Depression

Fecal transplants aren't what you think! Scientists are not harvesting the contents of local sewers to create a population of healthy bacteria. According to the Cleveland Clinic, volunteer fecal donors provide stool samples for fecal transplants. Healthcare providers rigorously screen volunteers before accepting them as fecal donors. They make sure the donor stool is free of any infections or diseases. After collecting the stool, they send it to a lab for processing. Fecal donations are blended with sterile saline and filtered, producing a liquid solution. The liquid might be used immediately, primarily if it's meant for someone. If not, it goes to a donor bank. The sample might be frozen to be thawed later or freeze-dried and put into capsules. Currently, two manufacturers in the United States produce these capsules for clinical use.

Fecal transplants are highly effective in treating a severe gastrointestinal disorder called *C. difficile*, which is caused by an overgrowth of toxic bacteria as the result of antibiotic overuse. A study published in the *New England Journal of Medicine* reported a success rate of over 80 percent.

Gut dysbiosis is involved in the development of an autoimmune disorder, systemic lupus, which we discuss in Chapter 12. In a twelve-week trial of fecal microbiota transplantation (FMT) in patients with active lupus, no adverse side effects were reported, and patients showed a significant decrease in symptoms from baseline.

FMT is being explored as a potential treatment for depression in humans, particularly in cases where traditional antidepressant therapy has been ineffective. Restoring a healthy gut microbiome through FMT may improve mental health, potentially by influencing the gut-brain axis.

In animal studies, rats subjected to chronic unpredictable mild stress and treated with FMT showed elevated brain levels of neurochemicals like serotonin, gamma-aminobutyric acid (GABA), and brain derived neurotrophic factor (BDNF), along with reduced inflammatory markers, leading to an alleviation of depressive symptoms. Similarly, after receiving gut microbiota from healthy donors, rats with depressive-like behaviors experienced significant improvement, highlighting FMT's capacity to influence mood regulation. Preclinical trials showed that germ-free adult rodents receiving fecal samples from human patients with depression showed increased depressive-like like behavior compared to controls. FMT aims to introduce a beneficial microbial gut community by transferring intestinal microbiota from a healthy donor to an affected patient.

A 2020 article published in *BMC Psychiatry* reported that in their review of eleven studies using FMT in depressed patients, all of the affected patients showed improvement in their depressive symptoms after administration of oral FMT capsules. A 2022 report describes a trial of FMT as an adjunctive therapy in depressed outpatients at a mood disorder clinic in Switzerland. The first patient had a diagnosis of major depression starting in adolescence with a suicide attempt later in life. She had two inpatient psychiatric hospitalizations and suffered from chronic constipation.

The second patient also had a history of major depression along with two psychiatric hospitalizations. She also suffered from chronic gastrointestinal symptoms. Both patients had already been treated with long-term therapy and a series of antidepressants without much improvement in their symptoms. Each patient was given frozen FMT capsules over the course of ninety minutes. The donors for the contents of the capsules were different for each subject, but each donor was depression free.

Within four weeks, both symptomatic patients had significant declines in their depressive symptoms without any side effects from the treatment. In addition, each had overall improvements in their gastrointestinal symptoms.

You Are What You Eat: The Link Between Diet and Mood

Did you know that your diet can affect your mood? One of the primary roles of the gut is to process and digest nutrients. What you eat directly influences the makeup of bacteria in your gut, which impacts your health. A healthy gut helps prevent chronic diseases like heart disease and cancer and reduces inflammation. A healthy gut keeps your brain healthy and enables you to maintain a healthy weight. Here is a quiz to test your knowledge of healthy and unhealthy ways to maintain a positive gut biome.

Which of the following can positively affect your gut health?

1. Eating fermented foods like sauerkraut and kimchi
2. Eating Jerusalem artichokes
3. Having a cocktail before dinner
4. Eating three meals per day
5. Having bacon and eggs for breakfast
6. Indulging in dark chocolate
7. Eating garlic

You are very gut savvy if you answered 1, 2, 4, 6, and 7. Studies found that heavy alcohol consumption changes your intestinal microbiome. However, research is lacking on the effect of moderate alcohol consumption on gut bacteria and how some elements in red wine interact with the gut. If you enjoy drinking, do so in moderation: one drink per day for women and two for men. The effect of moderate alcohol consumption on the gut microbiome is complex and may be beneficial in some instances, such as with red wine, where polyphenols may increase gut microbial diversity. However, alcohol can also negatively affect the gut by promoting dysbiosis (imbalance), potentially reducing beneficial bacteria, increasing detrimental ones, and even contributing to a weakened intestinal barrier or leaky gut.

Probiotics contain good bacteria and can be found in fermented foods like sauerkraut, kimchi, miso, and yogurt. Jerusalem artichokes contain a fiber that feeds the healthy bacteria in your gut. Processed foods like bacon, while tasting good, lack diversity and fiber. They are often filled with additives such as sugars, salt, or artificial sweeteners, contributing to poor gut health. This is not to say you can never have bacon, but try to eat it in moderation. Garlic isn't only good for keeping vampires at bay. It acts like preventative medicine and may reduce your risk of heart disease. It is an anti-inflammatory food and contains two healthy fibers. Dark chocolate is a rich source of antioxidants and minerals, and it generally contains less sugar than milk chocolate. Some research suggests that dark chocolate may help lower your risk of heart disease, reduce inflammation and insulin resistance, and improve your brain function.

You can also find probiotic supplement capsules. They have their advantages because you can selectively target the specific type of bacteria you want to ingest. They are usually also allergen free and contain no sugar. The literature generally promotes using supplements *and* eating probiotic foods for ultimate gut health.

Nutrient deficiency is implicated in the development of depression. These include omega-3 fatty acids, vitamin B, folate, vitamin D, zinc, and magnesium. Literature on nutrients in psychiatric illness has focused more on nutrient patterns than individual foods. For example, studies have repeatedly found that "traditional" or whole-food dietary patterns are correlated with less depression than those that Western societies typically follow. One pattern often cited as positively affecting mood is the Mediterranean diet, which is rich in seafood, fruits, vegetables, and grains.

In 2018, the *World Journal of Psychiatry* published the results of its study analyzing food nutrients to arrive at an Antidepressant Food Score (AFS), designed to identify the most nutrient-dense individual foods to prevent and promote recovery from depressive disorders and symptoms. To develop the AFS, a sample was gathered for a 100-gram serving of each food in raw form because cooking methods can alter food's nutrient bioavailability and water content. In addition, nutrients vary greatly in bioavailability and form between plant and animal foods. The mean antidepressant nutrient density was calculated for each food included. This generated a nutrient density score, which was expressed as a percentage for each type of food studied.

Antidepressant Animal-Based Food

Oyster 56%, Fish roe 19%

Lobster 17%, Emu 16%

Snapper 16%, Crab 24%

Clams 30%, Herring 16%

Salmon 10–16%, Goat 23%

Snail or whelk 16%, Smelt 20%

Liver and organ meats (spleen, kidneys, or heart) 18%–38%

Tuna 15%–21%

Poultry giblets 31%, Bluefish 19%

Mussels, Spot fish 16%, Wolffish 19%

Pollock 18%

Antidepressant Plant Foods

Watercress 127%, Pumpkin 46%, Kohlrabi 41%

Cauliflower 41%–42%, Red cabbage 41%, Broccoli 41%

Butternut squash 34% Papaya 31%, Lemon 31%

Strawberry 31%, Dandelion greens 43%, Brussels sprouts 35%

Acerola 34%

Spinach 97%

Mustard, turnip, or beet greens 76%–93%

Lettuces (red, green, romaine) 74%–99%

Swiss chard 90%

Fresh herbs 73%–75%

Chicory greens 74%

Peppers (bell, serrano, or jalapeno) 39%–56%

Kale or collards 48%–62%

Diet is crucial in discussing depression and anxiety because gut health is increasingly understood as critical for brain health. Generally, fiber is lacking in Western diets, influencing the population and diversity of bacterial species that make up the microbiome. Modifying behavior, such as dietary choices, is one way to alter one's genetic predisposition to disease.

Steps You Can Take to Create a Healthy Biome

- Eat a wide range of foods, mainly fruits and vegetables, that contribute to diversity in your gut.
- Eat fermented foods such as yogurt, sauerkraut, tempeh, and kefir, which are good sources of healthy bacteria.
- To lower inflammation, eat foods high in polyphenols (plant compounds), such as almonds, green tea, and dark chocolate.
- Limit artificial sweeteners, which hurt blood sugar and insulin response, and negatively affect your gut biome.
- Consider adding a probiotic supplement to your diet.
- Maintain a regular sleep routine. One study demonstrated that microbiome diversity improved with sleep efficiency and total sleep time and was negatively affected by sleep fragmentation.

MENDS Approach to Managing Gut Health and Psychiatric Symptoms

Medication. Many studies show that probiotics, particularly *Lactobacillus*, can prevent and manage several psychiatric disorders by modulating the gut biome. Nearly 30 percent of people with depression are drug-resistant. However, one researcher reported an enhanced patient response to antidepressants when it was combined with a probiotic. One research study reported that several of these types of probiotics changed the levels of neurotransmitters in an area of the brain in animal studies and alleviated depression-type behaviors. In humans, a study conducted in New Zealand of postpartum women with depression improved when they consumed a probiotic containing this type of bacteria. In adults, *L. acidophilus* has most often been taken orally, alone or with other probiotics, in doses of up to 60 billion CFUs daily for up to six months.

Exercise. Regular physical activity has been shown to influence the gut microbiome positively and may improve mood by increasing the production of mood-enhancing neurotransmitters and reducing inflammation. According to Dr. Christine Lee, gastroenterologist at the Cleveland Clinic, exercise is "probably the best 'medicine' we have for your gut." Exercise improves the gut biome in several ways. Your digestive tract is a muscle; like all muscles, it must be worked to stay healthy. If you remain inactive, the muscles in your gut that help digest food also become less active. Exercise improves circulation throughout your body, and it helps your gut remain stronger and able to maintain the appropriate balance of healthy bacteria. It also prevents constipation and bloating. Dr. Lee recommends thirty minutes of exercise, five days a week.

Nutrition. Try to follow a Mediterranean diet. It includes an abundance of fruits, vegetables, and whole grains. Consult the antidepressant food scale in this chapter and try incorporating some of the options that help improve mood. Carbohydrates are linked to serotonin, one of your essential neurotransmitters. However, choose your carbs wisely. Limit sugary foods and instead aim for complex carbs like whole grains. Make sure to include enough protein in your diet. Foods like turkey, tuna, and chicken contain an amino acid called tryptophan, a serotonin building block. Vegetarians and vegans can meet their protein needs by eating a variety of protein-rich plant foods, including legumes (beans, lentils, peas), soy products (tofu, tempeh, edamame), nuts, and seeds, along with whole grains like quinoa. Many protein powders are vegan.

Dhyana. Chronic stress can negatively affect your gut microbiome. Stress-reduction techniques like mindfulness, yoga, meditation, or deep breathing exercises can help improve your gut health and mood. A study published in 2023 in *General Psychiatry* found that a group of Tibetan Buddhist monks who practiced meditation daily had a different variety of gut microbes than their secular neighbors and were at lower risk for cardiovascular disease, depression, and anxiety.

Sleep. Sleeplessness and gut dysbiosis can be linked to inflammation. Insufficient sleep causes your body to produce more stress hormones, which can lead to cravings for unhealthy food choices like fat and sugar. It can also increase gut permeability. Sleep deprivation also increases your chances of developing reflux or indigestion.

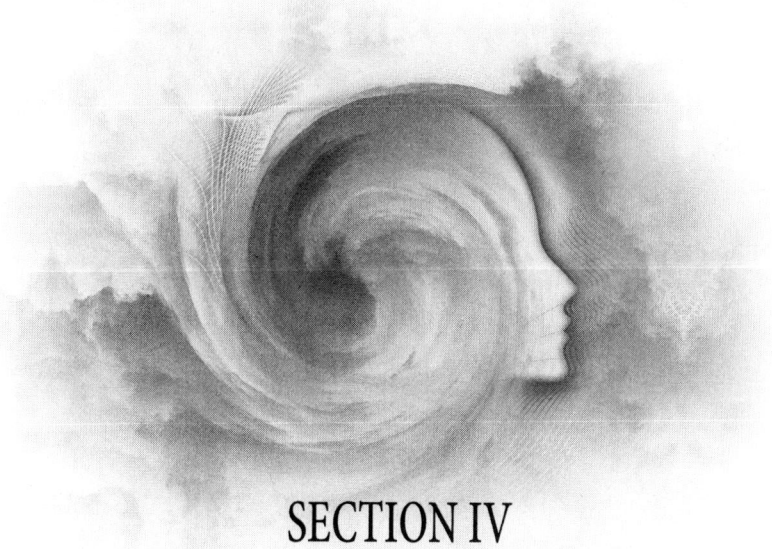

SECTION IV

•••

SNEAKY DISEASES AND PSYCHIATRIC SYMPTOMS

CHAPTER 7

CAN COVID CAUSE PSYCHIATRIC SYMPTOMS?

*We're learning so much about the virus daily
and how it can impact us in ways we might not expect.*
—JONATHAN LEWIN, executive VP for health affairs;
executive director, Woodruff Health Sciences Center, Emory University

Are you one of the millions of people who contracted COVID? If so, you understand the physical symptoms that made you feel miserable for days or even weeks. However, you might have continued to feel fatigued, unmotivated, tearful, irritable, and sad, even after the physical symptoms were gone. Living through a global pandemic was indeed hard on our mental health, even if we didn't get COVID, but researchers believe being depressed is not just the result of feeling sick, isolated, or fearing for our health or that of our loved ones. COVID-19 can produce changes in your brain that cause psychiatric symptoms.

Celia sought my help after her primary care physician could not explain her new onset of anxiety. Celia is a bright, attractive woman who works in a stressful, demanding job. She is married and has two small children.

"How can I help?" I asked after she sat down in my office.

"I'm not sure what is wrong with me. I have seen my primary care doctor, who referred me to a cardiologist."

"Can you fill me in a bit more? Why were you referred to a cardiologist?"

"It all started soon after I got my last COVID vaccination. My latest shot was from a different manufacturer than my first two shots. I didn't initially have any side effects, but within three or four months, I started having a racing heart for no apparent reason. It would just come on like out of nowhere. It felt like my heart was pounding out of my chest. Then, once or twice, I fainted after standing up from a chair. I am exhausted because I'm not sleeping well and feel nervous, but mostly before bed. My primary care doctor felt like I might have developed an arrhythmia, you know, like an irregular heartbeat, so that is why I had a consultation."

"Did he or she find anything wrong?"

"I had a full workup, an EKG, stress test, and I wore a monitor all the time for like a week, I think. All of it came back normal. So I went on with my life, which is always stressful. My job demands a lot of me, and I always like to do my best. It's hard being a working mom, but my kids are great, and my husband helps a lot. Then after all this, I had my first bout of COVID."

"How did this recent illness impact your symptoms?" I asked.

"They got worse."

Celia had no prior history of depression or anxiety and described herself as a generally upbeat person. She had no other medical issues. Her family history was only positive for anxiety in her older sister. Her marriage was stable, and she was secure in her professional life.

Although her cardiologist could not find anything unusual, he recommended she start on Propranolol. This medication is used for high blood pressure and also to decrease heart rate. Celia did not feel like it was doing much, so she returned to her primary care doctor, who suggested she start on a low dose of an antidepressant to treat what the doctor believed was an anxiety disorder. Before starting this medication, Sarah wanted to meet with me to see if I agreed with the recommendation.

Scientists have learned a great deal about COVID-19 and how it passes from one person to another, yet we don't know how the virus impacts our brain and other organs. The emergence of COVID-19 in late 2019 and its subsequent worldwide spread required the rapid development and implementation of vaccines to mitigate the pandemic's impact. By early January 2024, approximately 70.6 percent of the global population had received at least one vaccine dose. Although the efficacy of these vaccines in reducing severe illness, hospitalizations, and deaths has been well documented, the extensive vaccination campaigns have also led to research into the potential adverse side effects and, in some, the development of long COVID.

A 2024 study in *BMC Cardiovascular Disorders* looked at one of these side effects, known as the postural orthostatic tachycardia syndrome (POTS), which has been diagnosed in 2 to 14 percent of people following a COVID-19 infection. This long string of unfamiliar words means that some people develop problems with their autonomic nervous system. In people who develop POTS, some or all of these functions become dysfunctional. Think of your autonomic nervous system like a computer. Things run well without you noticing until something goes haywire, caused by a corrupted file—in this case, POTS. Usually, your blood pressure and heart rate fluctuate with posture. For example, when you get up from lying down, your blood pressure drops, and your heart rate increases to compensate. POTS sufferers, however, experience an abnormal autonomic response to an upright posture, causing fluctuating blood pressure readings and an increased heart rate. Increased heart rate and feelings of palpitations can occur in psychiatric conditions such as anxiety but also overlap with the profile of symptoms seen in patients with POTS. It is still unclear if this is due to a high prevalence of anxiety as a coexisting condition or if there is just an overlap of symptoms between the two conditions.

Investigators in this study reviewed all available global medical literature related to the development of POTS after a COVID-19 vaccine or infection. After extensive review, they concluded that "while an elevated risk of developing POTS exists following COVID-19 vaccination, the absolute risk remains significantly lower than that associated with infection." Most cases documented POTS symptom onset within days to a few weeks—up to three months after COVID-19 vaccination. Based on these patterns, POTS cases emerging within three months of vaccination are considered potentially related to the vaccine's ability to stimulate an immune response. The clinical presentations of POTS following COVID-19 vaccination are typically characterized by persistent increased heart rate, dizziness, fatigue, and palpitations, often emerging within two weeks after vaccine administration. This fit Celia's scenario very well.

The researchers describe some treatment modalities recommended for patients with severe symptoms. Sometimes this requires treatment with steroids or a medication called Ivabradine, which is used to treat patients with heart failure. For those with POTS, this drug helps lower their heart rate without lowering their blood pressure. Other treatment recommendations include lifestyle changes such as wearing compression stockings to maintain blood pressure and increasing salt and water intake. Mostly, the treatment must be tailored to each patient's individual needs.

Celia's case was a bit more complex because her physical symptoms were likely caused by the vaccine or the actual infection, or both, leading to the development of an unwanted conditioned response. Even though there were many times she was not experiencing the physical symptoms, the fact that they mainly occurred before bed led to the development of a paradigm where an innocuous event (going to bed) became paired with a feared response. A conditioned response is a learned behavior that combines a potent stimulus (racing heart) with a neutral one (going to bed).

Here's an example: Remember when you were a child and sometimes going to the doctor meant getting an injection? (I certainly do!) You may have developed a fear of going to the doctor for any reason, even if it was for a benign reason like your school physical.

According to a 2023 review in *Cureus,* anxiety is a common symptom seen in POTS and other autonomic disorders. The authors suggest that anxiety develops due to either excessive awareness and apprehension of physical symptoms related to fluctuating blood pressure or a conditioned fear response resulting in an increased heart rate when individuals resume an upright position.

Celia's self-described anxious feelings were causing insomnia and were related to her daytime fatigue. The propranolol her cardiologist prescribed was helping with the incidents of rapid heart rate and fluctuating blood pressure, but she was still anxious. She did not have any symptoms of depression, so I did not think she needed an antidepressant. Instead, I prescribed a low dose of clonazepam. This type of medicine decreases anxiety and lasts long enough to help her relax, fall asleep, and hopefully sleep through the night.

People with POTS naturally wonder about when it will go away. According to the American Academy of Family Physicians, many patients spontaneously recover within twelve months. A study in the *Journal of General and Family Medicine* reports their findings after following thirty-two patients with COVID-19-induced POTS for up to 159 days. In this study, many patients with POTS had psychiatric symptoms caused by financial and educational concerns because of their inability to go to work or attend school, and anxiety about prolonged symptoms. They stated that in many patients, the symptoms improved over time, such that they could return to work or school. However, in a different study, only 33 out of 172 subjects had complete resolution of their symptoms after five years.

Although the pandemic began over five years ago, before I started writing this book, COVID-19 is still considered a new illness, so it is not surprising that research has limited information on what can be expected regarding the duration of unwanted side effects or symptoms.

Depression is a medical condition whose cause is often multifactorial. Symptoms of depression include low energy, loss of interest in usual activities, decreased appetite, poor sleep, and low mood. These are also seen in people suffering from COVID.

A recent study in *The Lancet* reported that persistent depression and anxiety can follow severe cases of COVID-19. However, it appears that depression following a bout with this illness is not only a lingering effect of having felt miserable. The isolation and hospitalization that many faced, as well as the fear of death, are significant stressors. When stressed, your body turns on its autonomic nervous system. The portion of this system that lights up in an emergency is the sympathetic nervous system, which prepares you for fight-or-flight. This results in your body's initiation of an inflammatory response, which is a central theory that explains how infections such as COVID lead to psychiatric illness.

In 2018, British psychiatrist Edward Bullmore published a book titled *The Inflamed Mind*. He postulates that depression and other mental illnesses could be the result of immune system activation. Researchers previously believed the brain had an impenetrable wall known as the blood-brain barrier. However, we now know that open channels exist between the brain and immune system elements. Bullmore argues that when inflammation occurs, cytokines cross the BBB, leading to changes within the brain that result in depression. Cytokines appear to instigate depression by impacting the brain's neurotransmitters, causing their levels to drop below healthy concentrations. Studies have consistently found higher levels of inflammatory proteins in patients with major depressive disorder.

In 2020, researchers studied over four hundred COVID survivors who sought treatment at an emergency room and found that, overall, over 50 percent scored in the unhealthy range for psychiatric symptoms. This included depression, anxiety, post-traumatic stress disorder, and obsessive-compulsive disorder. Of the patients studied, those more likely to develop these symptoms included women, patients with a preexisting psychiatric diagnosis, and those who had previously managed their COVID symptoms at home. On follow-up three months later, at least one-third of those studied still experienced psychiatric symptoms in at least one area.

Long-term symptoms associated with COVID-19 are collectively known as *long COVID-19*. A 2022 review article in the *Journal of Psychiatric Research* reported current findings in a series of studies that looked at neuropsychiatric complications of long COVID in adults, which resembles chronic fatigue syndrome.

The most common complaints include severe incapacitating fatigue, pain, compromised sleep, and cognitive difficulties. Cognitive impairment is more frequently observed in patients who require admission to the ICU. Similar to findings reported in 2020, the main risk factors for depression in these studies included being a female with a previous psychiatric history.

Unfortunately, unlike other complaints, psychiatric symptoms were slow to resolve and sometimes lasted more than twelve months. The authors reviewed several studies examining changes in brain metabolism and anatomy after a COVID infection. One study reported the results of patient PET scans (a technique that measures physiological function by looking at blood flow and metabolism) three weeks after a COVID infection. They found decreased metabolism in several brain areas, and interestingly, brain fog was correlated with highly specific regions of reduced metabolism.

In a different study that looked at MRI images of participants after infection, researchers found that the severity of depression that patients reported was correlated with the degree of decreased volume in an area of the brain associated with emotions and behavior. The authors of both studies concluded that brain inflammation during an acute episode of COVID predicted structural and functional changes in survivors' brains, as well as psychiatric complications in those with long COVID.

In patients with COVID, serotonin may work to prevent or limit the cytokine release process that is partly responsible for worsening the inflammatory component of the illness. In this way, serotonin may also have some ability to decrease pain, as well as the formation of blood clots, which is one of the risks of severe COVID-19 infection and often leads to death.

Antidepressants are often prescribed for patients with depression to increase the brain's level of neurotransmitters. A preliminary study using antidepressants to treat patients with COVID who had coexisting depressive symptoms showed rapid improvement in reports of depressive symptoms—within four weeks. In addition, a fascinating secondary effect of using SSRIs also showed promise in decreasing the inflammatory properties of the virus itself. Blocking reuptake makes more serotonin available to help pass messages between brain cells.

In the fall of 2021, Canadian scientists published a study using fluvoxamine, an SSRI, in nearly 1,500 Brazilian patients with chronic illnesses who were recently infected with the coronavirus. Half of the patients took the antidepressant at home for ten days; the rest received a sugar pill. Participants were followed for four weeks to determine who required hospitalization or spent extended time in an emergency room when hospitals were full. In the group that took the drug, 11 percent needed hospitalization or an extended ER stay, compared to 16 percent of those on the placebo. The results published in *Lancet Global Health* were so strong that independent experts monitoring the study recommended stopping it early because the results were clear.

A month later, a University of California–San Francisco/Stanford research group published its work analyzing electronic health records from an extensive database, which had information from almost 500,000 patients across the United States. This included 83,584 adult patients diagnosed with COVID-19 between January and September 2020. Of those, 3,401 patients were prescribed two SSRIs, fluoxetine and fluvoxamine. The results showed that patients taking fluoxetine were 28 percent less likely to die, those taking either fluoxetine or fluvoxamine were 26 percent less likely to die, and the entire group of patients taking any kind of SSRI was 8 percent less likely to die than the matched patient controls.

The treatment of long COVID is dynamic and multidisciplinary, depending on the involved systems and the patient's relative signs and symptoms. According to an article in the *Nepal Journal of Epidemiology*, a large proportion of individuals reportedly seek self-care and often resort to a combination of medications to gain relief from the worst symptoms. Although no single treatment is recommended for patients who experience neuropsychiatric symptoms after COVID, the American Academy of Physical Medicine and Rehabilitation Multi-Disciplinary Post-COVID Collaborative published a guidance statement specifically focused on the cognitive-related symptoms that can occur in people who have been diagnosed with acute COVID-19 infection or were presumed to have had the infection and initially experienced mild to severe symptoms. Their recommendations included the following:

- For patients who screen positive for cognitive symptoms, referral to a specialist with expertise in formal cognitive assessment and remediation, such as a neuropsychologist.
- Treat, in collaboration with appropriate specialists, underlying medical conditions, such as pain, insomnia/sleep disorders, and mood disorders that may be contributing to

cognitive symptoms. This may include referral to a psychiatrist or mental health specialist.
- Complete, in collaboration with the patient's primary care provider, medication polypharmacy reduction. The goal is to wean or eliminate medications if medically feasible, with an emphasis on drugs that may impact cognition.
- Reinforce sleep hygiene techniques, including nonpharmacologic approaches, which could mean cognitive behavioral methods to reset the sleep cycle.
- Patients should be advised to begin an individualized, structured, titrated return to activity. For patients who achieve a return to their normal daily activities, regular exercise (at least two to three times per week of aerobic exercise) may be effective in improving cognition and contributing to improved sleep patterns.
- Ensure frequent assessment of the impact of "return to normal." Daily activities are recommended to ensure that symptoms do not flare, and that exercise is tolerated.

CHAPTER 8

LYME DISEASE: THE GREAT IMITATOR

*I learned what it is like to have a disease with
no diagnosis, to be baffled by what insurance covers and
what it does not, and to have a mind that can't think
fast enough to know whether a red traffic light
means to press on the gas or hit the brakes.*
—AMY TAN

Amy Tan, the bestselling author of *The Joy Luck Club*, is not one of my patients. However, I often use her story when speaking about the neuropsychiatric symptoms caused by Lyme disease and how frequently they are missed or misinterpreted. Her history is all too familiar to those seeking help for puzzling symptoms, so I thought it would be helpful to examine it in this chapter. At the end of this section, I include a link to a YouTube video in which Tan gives a firsthand account of her experience.

In July 1999, Amy Tan attended a wedding in upstate New York. It was an outdoor event in a venue surrounded by trees and a babbling brook. The following day, she saw a bright red rash on her shin. She thought briefly about Lyme but believed her rash was not the classic bull's-eye lesion described in the literature. Instead, the rash had a black speck in the center, so Tan believed it was a spider bite. Over time, the rash grew larger and brighter in color. After a month, she developed red splotches on her arms. In addition to the rash, she had developed symptoms similar to the flu. However, she was not alarmed because the symptoms disappeared within a day.

In the years that followed, Tan experienced headaches, insomnia, muscle aches, fatigue, and jitteriness. At her annual physical, she told her primary care doctor about tingling and numbness in her feet. He explained she had neuropathy, a medical term that describes damage or disease of the nerves, particularly those outside the brain and spinal cord, but did not explain why this should exist. Tan told him about her history of a rash and asked whether all of her symptoms might be related. "No," her doctor replied, dismissing her concerns.

In search of an answer, the author visited multiple specialists. She told her husband she believed something in her body was "broken." At one point, her blood sugar plunged so low when she checked it at home that her doctor recommended hospitalization. During the hospitalization, an MRI of her brain showed fourteen abnormal lesions. Her doctors told her, "It's normal for someone your age." At the time, she was forty-nine.

An incidental finding on a scan of her adrenal gland led to

surgery, which unfortunately was complicated by a surgical error, requiring a much more complicated procedure. After surgery, Tan started taking steroids, and her symptoms briefly improved, only to become more severe and bizarre. She started hallucinating, seeing images of little girls, poodles hanging upside down, and brightly lit odometers. She experienced unpleasant smells and developed seizures. Her memory was poor, and her concentration waned. When she wrote, she reversed numbers and substituted inaccurate words. She became lost in the neighborhood where she had lived for over thirty years.

The physicians whom Tan consulted were experts in their fields and affiliated with major medical centers. They never raised the idea that she was creating her symptoms, but they also never considered Lyme as the diagnosis. As a result, she was never tested for it. Her doctors told her the likelihood that she had Lyme was very small because she lived in California, where Lyme disease was not prevalent. However, she reminded her doctors that she also had a home in upstate New York, but again, her concerns were dismissed.

At one point, she was given an ELISA test, one of the initial screening tests for the type of bacteria that causes Lyme and other disorders. It came back negative. She asked about the accuracy of the test and was told she hadn't been tested for Lyme, but for another disorder caused by the same type of bacteria: syphilis! Lyme disease is caused by a bacteria called a *spirochete* (the same type of bacteria that causes syphilis). So she didn't have syphilis, but what did she have?

After months of searching for answers, Tan conducted her own internet research and read about the lack of accuracy of ELISA tests, particularly in individuals with late-stage Lyme. She found a doctor with expertise in treating patients with Lyme disease who confirmed her diagnosis with a more specific test. After a course of antibiotics, she began to feel better, but it took almost two years for her to feel well. Despite this, as she recounts firsthand, she has residual symptoms because it took so long to receive appropriate care.

What Is Lyme Disease and Why Is a Psychiatrist Writing About It?

The first mention of this disorder in the medical literature was in 1883 in Europe, when a German doctor described the classic rash in one of his patients. Nearly forty years later, a French doctor linked the rash in one of his patients to a recent tick bite.

In the United States, Lyme disease was named after a town in Connecticut where it was first diagnosed in children in 1975 and believed to be a variant of juvenile rheumatoid arthritis. Many psychiatrists see patients with documented or suspected Lyme disease because of the significant overlap in symptoms between Lyme disease and common psychiatric disorders such as anxiety, depression, obsessive-compulsive disorder, mania, psychosis, and, most worrisome, suicidal thoughts. The *American Journal of Psychiatry* published the results of an extensive Danish study in 2021. To conduct their study, the researchers analyzed the medical records of nearly 7 million people living in Denmark over twenty-two years. They compared the mental health data of individuals after a hospital-based diagnosis of Lyme disease to the rest of the Danish population who had never had a Lyme diagnosis recorded in the medical register. Patients who had a history of mental disorder or suicidality before the Lyme disease diagnosis were excluded from the analysis. According to the authors, the rate of mood disorders was highest during the first year after a Lyme diagnosis, and highest for completed suicide within the first three years.

A study conducted in 2004 at Columbia University's Lyme and Tick-Borne Disease Research Center found children with Lyme disease had substantial cognitive and psychiatric disturbances, and neuropsychiatric symptoms may be the first ones recognized, or they can surface months or even years later, like Amy Tan's did. The bacteria, *Borrelia burgdorferi*, is transmitted by deer ticks. Lyme disease bacteria can cause a wide array of symptoms. It is commonly associated with the classic bull's-eye lesion. However, most affected individuals do not recall being bitten by a tick. The following image illustrates the classic bull's-eye lesion:

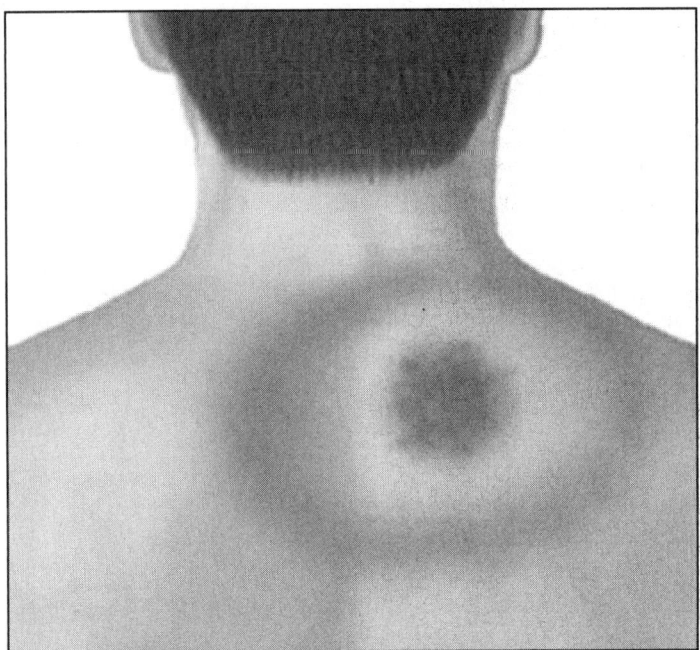

Fig. 8.1 Classic Lyme Bull's-Eye Lesion

What Are the Symptoms of Lyme Disease and Why Is It Often Misdiagnosed?

Most people infected with *B. burgdorferi* experience one or more clinical signs of Lyme disease. Similar to many other infections caused by these types of bacteria, the clinical manifestations of Lyme disease occur in different phases, each capable of remission and exacerbation of symptoms. Due to the varied nature of the symptoms and because they may worsen or improve, it is easy to see why patients with this diagnosis are often dismissed or misdiagnosed, especially if the classic target lesion is absent, or the individual does not live in an area known to be a hot spot for Lyme. Infection with the bacteria occurs in stages, and depending on when an individual seeks care, the history and physical presentation may appear quite differently, adding to the confusion for the patient and the medical provider.

The first part of early infection is called the localized stage and is recognized by an expanding red skin lesion at the site of the tick bite. Approximately 75 percent of people who experience the rash develop it within thirty days. However, due to the small size of the tick and the lack of pain or itching at the site, only about one-third of those affected will recall having been bitten.

The second stage of early Lyme disease begins shortly after the initial stage. The bacteria spreads through the bloodstream, where it can affect distant organs. During this stage, varied symptoms begin, and the clinical presentation mimics various illnesses, leading to possible misdiagnosis. One-half of infected individuals develop a more widespread rash. Facial rashes sometimes occur. Combined with other symptoms such as fever, chills, headache, and joint and muscle aches, this often leads to suspicion of an autoimmune disorder.

Left untreated or misdiagnosed, Lyme can affect various organ systems. Recall Tan's history of seizures, confusion, and ultimately hallucinations from the effect of the disease on her brain. Late-stage Lyme disease can produce unrelenting arthritis and, in rare cases, a disfiguring skin condition. Given the sometimes-confusing presentation of this disease, as well as an often-misleading history, how is it correctly diagnosed?

Diagnosis of Lyme Disease

In the 1990s, in an effort to improve specificity, the Centers for Disease Control and Prevention (CDC) adopted a two-tiered testing strategy. We've discussed the first test: ELISA. If this is negative, no further testing is recommended. A second test called the Western blot should be ordered if the result is equivocal or positive. A positive Western blot could show an elevation of one or more antibodies, called IgM or IgG. If exposure to ticks is recent, and a positive IgM or IgG result is detected, there is good evidence that a recent infection occurred. If the infection is greater than four weeks old, and a positive IgG result is present, this is good evidence of a current or previous infection. Because the IgM tests are less specific than the IgG-based tests, the CDC recommends using only IgG results if the infection is over four weeks old.

Early magnetic resonance imaging (MRI) studies of acute neurologic Lyme disease showed white matter changes in the brains of those with the disease, like those seen with Amy Tan. SPECT brain imaging, which assesses blood flow, shows areas of decreased perfusion, which in some patients improves or disappears after appropriate antibiotic treatment. Interestingly, in some studies, the pattern seen looks much like the one in patients with the autoimmune disorder lupus.

Why Is There Confusion Around Diagnosis?

Tests for the detection of antibodies to Lyme disease are not perfect. They depend on several factors, such as the time it takes for detectable antibody levels to be produced by your body, as well as the quality of the method used to detect them. Sometimes, if the test is given too soon after a tick bite, the initial test may return negative because your immune system has not had enough time to develop antibodies. Two-stage testing has limited sensitivity during an early infection but has excellent sensitivity in people infected for several weeks. The limited sensitivity of antibody tests during early infection is not considered a problem in most cases because the diagnosis of Lyme disease at this point is confirmed clinically by recognizing the characteristic skin lesion.

Even in cases where a rash was not detected or was atypical, antibodies should be detectable during recovery, a few weeks after the initial phase. Despite these recognized limitations, antibody detection following the CDC guidelines performs well for most people with objective symptoms consistent with Lyme disease, other than a bull's-eye lesion.

There is controversy regarding individuals who are experiencing chronic, poorly defined clinical syndromes who have tested negative using validated tests for the detection of antibodies to *B. burgdorferi*. Some individuals seeking a diagnosis for their symptoms may encounter providers who use unconventional, nonvalidated testing methods. Unfortunately, several laboratories in the United States are offering these tests. Patients tested by these laboratories may be erroneously diagnosed as having Lyme disease and then may undergo long courses of unnecessary antibiotics. Unfortunately, the long-term use of antibiotics can lead to severe side effects, such as dysregulation of the gastric biome and, in rare cases, even death due to a bacterial overgrowth of *C. difficile*.

Why Is There Controversy over Treatment for Lyme Disease?

Despite the growing international incidence of Lyme disease, treatment has not attracted significant financial investment from pharmaceutical companies. In addition, the evidence-based and international guidelines for chronic Lyme treatment and management continue to be conflicting and controversial.

In general, the treatment recommendation is a two- to four-week course of oral antibiotics, which is more successful in the early stages of the disease. The controversy surrounding Lyme treatment centers around whether the infection persists and causes chronic symptoms despite an appropriate course of antibiotics. Some researchers believe the persistence of symptoms is the result of an overreaction of the immune system to the Lyme infection, leading to a secondary autoimmune disorder, a crucial distinction. Persistent disease requires ongoing antibiotic treatment, which can be harmful if you do not have an active infection.

In general, if you are diagnosed with Lyme disease confirmed by laboratory testing, or if you have the presence of the classic rash, a two- to four-week course of antibiotic treatment should be curative. But what if you have symptoms that linger long after you receive standard antibiotic treatment?

Chronic Lyme disease is a poorly defined term applied to patients with persistent symptoms such as fatigue, muscle and joint pain, and mental fogginess that linger long after appropriate antibiotic treatment. In 2006, the Infectious Disease Society of America defined post-treatment Lyme disease syndrome (PTLDS) as a constellation of symptoms—including fatigue, cognitive dysfunction, or muscle aches—that result in disability and persist for at least six months after adequate treatment.

Researchers estimate that 10 to 20 percent of individuals diagnosed with Lyme disease and receiving appropriate treatment may have this syndrome. Several theories explain why these symptoms might continue for months or even years. Some of the bacteria might have the ability to evade your immune system. The bacterial residue could trigger chronic inflammation, as a previous chapter discussed. Another theory suggests that a severe infection, delayed treatment, or coinfection with an additional tick-borne bacteria could lead to an uncontrolled immune system overreaction.

The Centers for Disease Control and Prevention does not recognize post-treatment Lyme syndrome. Neither does the Infectious Diseases Society of America nor the American Academy of Neurology.

Alternative practitioners who are self-designated "Lyme-literate" often make this diagnosis, which at times can lead to unnecessary testing and an overuse of antibiotics, as well as supplements that they profess treat this disorder. Many patients in my practice with these symptoms have visited alternative providers. They arrive with a handful of test results that show clearly negative results on Western blot tests only to be told they have chronic Lyme disease and need lifelong treatment. One patient brought in a grocery bag full of medication bottles, some of which had no relation to treating an infectious disease. Another patient had a bottle of Ivermectin, which veterinarians use to treat dog parasites. Still another told me she was receiving hyperbaric oxygen several times a month for $500 per visit!

What can you do if you are experiencing symptoms after appropriate treatment for an evidence-based (two-step testing) case of Lyme disease? According to a 2023 study in *Antibiotics,* treatment should be based on the presumed cause of the disease. If persistent infection is suspected, repeated antibiotic therapy should be considered. In post-Lyme arthritis, for example, failure of one course of antibiotic treatment is often followed by a second.

Aside from antibiotics, some off-label pharmacologic treatments and nonpharmacologic therapies primarily focus on managing your symptoms and restoring or improving your overall functioning. For example, pregabalin and Cymbalta may provide some symptom improvement for chronic pain. Although the exact mechanism of action is unknown, these medications work by calming irritated, overactive nerves. Older antidepressants such as nortriptyline are often used for symptomatic management of pain and sleep. SSRIs may be indicated for managing secondary depression or anxiety.

In the same 2023 study, the authors proposed a different mechanism for treating post-Lyme symptoms (PTLDS)—vagus nerve stimulation. Recall, the vagus nerve is the main nerve of your parasympathetic nervous system (PNS), the part of your autonomic nervous system that counterbalances your sympathetic nervous system system (SNS). While your SNS prepares you for fight-or-flight, your PNS helps your body's response during rest. This system manages body functions such as digestion, heart rate, and breathing. In research studies, vagus nerve stimulation shows promise in improving mood and decreasing pain and inflammation.

Lyme disease and PTLDS are linked to inflammation. This novel approach may be valuable in some patients who do not respond well to antibiotics or prefer not to take medication. Preclinical trials with animals show that vagus nerve stimulation provides an anti-inflammatory effect.

In humans, vagus nerve stimulators are more effective if implanted rather than operated outside your body. The noninvasive form is newer and hasn't yet been proven consistently effective.

Nonpharmacologic interventions such as cognitive behavioral therapy (CBT) can help ease symptom burden and manage the stress of living with a chronic illness. Mindfulness-based stress reduction has been studied with patients who have fibromyalgia and shows promise in reducing symptoms of pain, fatigue, and stress levels. In one research study of individuals with persistent Lyme disease symptoms, a supervised resistance exercise program increased the number of days study participants reported feeling healthy and energetic.

So what can you do if you experience persistent symptoms of Lyme after appropriate antibiotic treatment?

- Consider a regular, supervised exercise program using weights or resistance bands.
- Ask your provider about the possibility of a trial of an antidepressant or pregabalin to reduce pain and improve your sleep.
- Consider working with a cognitive behavioral therapist or enrolling in a mindfulness-based stress reduction program. A free program is available at palousemindfulness.com.

In her own voice, Amy Tan describes her experience with undiagnosed Lyme at "Amy Tan Suffers Lyme Disease: A Genius Mind Goes Missing," YouTube, July 1, 2012, https://youtu.be/YMVbh03kAbY.

CHAPTER 9

EPSTEIN-BARR VIRUS: NOT JUST THE KISSING DISEASE

Elaine: "My roommate has Lyme disease."
Jerry: "I thought she had Epstein-Barr syndrome?"
Elaine: "She has this in addition to Epstein-Barr. It's like Epstein-Barr with a twist of Lyme disease."
—SEINFELD, May 16, 1991

Allie, a third-year undergraduate at an Ivy League university, came to my office one fall day while she was on medical leave. She was petite, dressed in jeans and a loose college sweatshirt, and had light brown hair cut in a short bob. Behind her oversized glasses were her striking, brilliant blue eyes.

"How can I help you, Allie?" I asked as she took a seat on my office couch.

"I don't know what's wrong with me. All I want to do is sleep. I sleep for eight hours, get up, and then want to go back to sleep. I can't think, and my brain is foggy. I worked so hard to get into this school, and now I'm afraid I will never be able to return, like something is wrong with my brain." At this point, Allie started to cry. When she composed herself, she told me this story:

I started at a state school, not because my parents couldn't afford a private school. I didn't want to be obligated to them, so I got a full academic scholarship to State. I was doing well there, made friends, and did extracurriculars like tutoring students in math. After a few years, I just got bored and had always wanted to attend an Ivy League school, so I applied as a transfer and got in.

Things were different there. Everyone was wealthy, or they came from a prep school. The other thing was that all the girls in my suite had eating disorders and weighed themselves constantly. All they talked about was how little they ate, and they were all in competition for who was the skinniest. I'm not fat by any means, but next to them, I looked enormous! Anytime we would go out for ice cream, at least one of them would take laxatives so she would drop some water weight before eating. After a while, it got to me.

I wasn't sleeping well. I was afraid to eat in front of them because I felt like they were constantly judging me. I liked my classes and was doing well, but it was hard to make friends since I transferred in as a junior.

The one good thing was that I met this guy. He is a lovely dental student. I've seen him several times. We haven't had sex yet, but we fooled around a little. Right around midterms, I got really sick. I had a sore throat and swollen glands. I thought it was just a virus and never skipped classes, so I continued, even while ill. I went to student health, and they told me it was probably just a virus, to take Tylenol. When my parents arrived for parents' weekend, I told them what was going on and couldn't stop crying. They were worried. I had lost so much weight and wasn't sleeping well, so we talked about taking a medical leave. I didn't want to do this, but I really could not function feeling as I did.

I slept for fourteen hours the first night I was home. I saw my primary care doctor, who did some blood work and said I didn't have strep, but I wonder if I have mono; several of my suitemates got it around the time I got sick. My doctor doubted it but agreed to do another blood test. Sure enough, it was positive. Sadly, there is nothing you can do for mono. You have to treat the symptoms. It has been several weeks, and I still have no energy, but more importantly, I feel sad and hopeless. I don't look forward to anything, and my mom has to remind me to eat. I thought I would feel better by now. I worked so hard to get into the school of my dreams, and now I wonder if I can ever return.

What Is Epstein-Barr, and How Does It Cause Depression?

Epstein-Barr virus (EBV) is the leading cause of infectious mononucleosis. It has been given the popular name the "kissing disease" because kissing is the primary route of transmission among adolescents and young adults. *Infectious mononucleosis*, or *glandular fever*, is a clinical diagnosis characterized by fever, sore throat, swollen glands, and often prolonged fatigue. The prolonged fatigue you may experience can mimic depressive symptoms, and infectious mononucleosis has been a suspected risk factor for developing depression for decades. Approximately 90 percent of infectious mononucleosis cases are caused by an EBV infection. EBV infections are so prevalent that approximately 90 percent of adults under the age of thirty have positive antibodies for the virus—meaning they either have a current, past, or latent (present but not causing symptoms) infection.

One of the most extensive research studies that looked at the association between infection with EBV and depression was completed in Denmark over an eighteen-year period. Researchers followed over 1 million individuals who tested positive for EBV after the age of ten and were later diagnosed with depression. The results indicated a 40 percent greater risk for developing depression after the first year of infection than for age-matched individuals who had never contracted the virus. The underlying biological mechanisms involved in the increased risk of depression after infectious mononucleosis are still unclear. However, inflammation and its effect on the immune system and brain function appear to be involved.

In 1998, University of California scientist Benjamin Hart proposed an animal model of depression resulting from infection with a pathogen. He injected an infectious agent into animals and observed their responses of decreased appetite, decreased grooming behavior, and low energy, like what is observed in humans who experience depression. When he reversed the infectious agent, the animal's behavior resolved. This contributed to our current understanding of how inflammation is the common link between the two disorders.

Karl A. Menninger was the first researcher to link influenza, a type of virus, with neuropsychiatry. Dr. Menninger reported his study of one hundred patients admitted to Boston area hospitals with behavioral changes that occurred in 1918 during the Spanish flu epidemic. Sven-Erik Mamelund studied psychiatric hospitalizations during the same period and found the number of first-time hospitalizations due to influenza-related mental disorders was seven times greater six years after the pandemic. The Spanish flu survivors reported sleep disturbances, depression, dizziness, and difficulty coping at work, and there were increased death rates due to suicide. These symptoms are also seen in individuals suffering from depression.

Research studies report that a protein created in the early phase of EBV replication can stimulate your immune system to produce pro-inflammatory proteins called cytokines. Cytokines are elevated in the blood of individuals who are experiencing depression, so the connection between infection with viruses such as EBV and mood disorders such as depression seems to be mediated by the inflammatory process. A mononucleosis infection can put you at a 40 percent greater risk for a depressive episode in the future. This virus can lie dormant in your body for your lifetime, but stress can reactivate it. In a Japanese study, researchers found that psychological stress was significantly associated with EBV reactivation in women. The researchers suggest that psychological stress can suppress your immune system, which allows the virus to reactivate.

What about Allie? Her diagnosis of mononucleosis, presumably due to EBV, was confirmed. Still, she was exhibiting many symptoms of depression, such as sleeping too much, poor appetite, low mood, feelings of hopelessness, and loss of interest in her usual activities.

She agreed to a trial of sertraline, a type of SSRI, and responded well within a few weeks. She stayed home for the remainder of the semester, then returned to school and graduated on time by taking extra classes. That would seem to be the end of the story—but it isn't. Allie and I would cross paths again ten years later when she was applying to medical school after completing a postbaccalaureate premed program and experiencing medically unexplained symptoms.

Does EBV Infection Explain Long COVID Symptoms?

About 30 percent of patients who have been infected with COVID-19 experience long-term symptoms following recovery from their acute illness: fatigue, brain fog, sleep difficulties, joint aches, pharyngitis, muscle aches, headaches, fever, gastrointestinal upset, and skin rashes.

As mentioned, approximately 90 percent of the global population has been infected by EBV, a type of herpes virus, by the time they reach adulthood. It can be sneaky and stay quiet or become active again and cause a reemergence of the symptoms commonly associated with mononucleosis. Many symptoms attributed to long COVID-19 are the same as, or very similar to, those associated with EBV reactivation. Scientists at a hospital in China were the first to document EBV reactivation in COVID-19 patients during the acute phase of illness. They found that more than half of hospitalized COVID-19 patients tested for EBV between January and February 2020 had lab tests indicating EBV reactivation within two weeks of testing positive for COVID-19. Scientists in Italy and France reported similar results.

A 2021 multisite study looked at 185 individuals with evidence of confirmed COVID-19 infections. Thirty percent of them reported long COVID-19 symptoms for at least thirty days after testing positive. They were compared with age-matched individuals who had not experienced COVID-19. The results showed that the study group had almost seven times the rate of positive blood tests indicating reactivation with EBV than the control group. Interestingly, EBV has been associated with tinnitus and hearing loss, which is a common long COVID-19 symptom, and was reported by seven subjects in the research study groups who tested positive for EBV reactivation.

Based on their results, the researchers concluded there is a likelihood that EBV reactivation occurs early in COVID-19 infection. They hypothesized that it is worth considering that a portion of long COVID-19 symptoms may result from COVID-19 inflammation-induced EBV reactivation.

The Connection Between Psychological Stress and Infectious Disease

The relationship between psychological stress and medical illness is complex. We each have our unique susceptibility to stress and how we manage it. Some factors that influence this include genetic vulnerability, coping style, personality type, and social support. However, not all stress has an adverse effect. Studies have shown that short-term stress can boost your immune system and can help athletes perform at their peak (*eustress*), but chronic stress (*distress*) can ultimately contribute to illness.

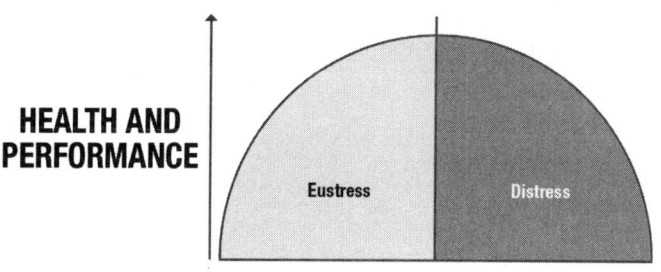

Fig. 9.1 Eustress Is the Action-Enhancing Stress That Give Athletes the Competitive Edge

A study linking psychosocial stress to illness defined *stress* as "a process in which environmental demands strain an organism's adaptive capacity, resulting in both psychological demands as well as biological changes that could increase the risk for illness." In Allie's case, she was enrolled at a prestigious university, felt the need to perform academically, and succumbed to the social pressure to be thin and "perfect" like her new friends. She deprived herself of adequate sleep, limited her food intake, and exercised excessively to fit in with her peers.

In some countries where hard work and long hours are the norm, there is an increased risk of suicide among workers. For example, Japan and China each have a word for death by overwork—*karoshi* and *guolaosi*. These countries recognize suicide as an official work-related condition. In the United Kingdom, the estimated prevalence of stress and stress-related conditions rose significantly from 1990 to 2002. In the last year the data were collected, over 13 million workdays were lost due to stress-related anxiety and depression. In the United States, psychological stress is an independent risk factor for serious illnesses such as heart disease, cancer, accidental injuries, gastrointestinal disorders, and suicide.

Several studies report that chronic stress compromises your body's ability to mount an immune response to an infectious agent. This is partly due to the surge in stress hormones produced under perceived duress.

Although no vaccine is available against the Epstein-Barr virus, there is much interest and research into how it can be treated or even prevented. In 2020, researchers at University of Utah Health discovered that EBV uses a novel strategy to survive in the human body. The virus takes hold of its host's cellular machinery to make copies of itself, prioritizing the production of its proteins over those of the host cell. In 2020, the same research team found that spironolactone, a medicine routinely used to treat heart failure, has an unexpected antiviral activity against EBV. They discovered that the drug targets an EBV protein, essential for viral replication.

In a recent National Institutes of Health study, investigators reported on a possible new way of treating and preventing EBV. They discovered a weak spot in the virus and attempted to target it with a new technology. EBV has a protein that it uses to infect a host's cells. Using an antibody developed to block this protein prevented the development of EBV infections in animal models. Ongoing studies will someday be applied to humans to prevent or lessen the course of this virus.

MENDS Approach to Managing Inflammation Due to Infection

Medication. A preliminary study using antidepressants to treat patients with COVID showed rapid improvement in reports of depressive symptoms. In addition, SSRI medications showed promise in reducing the inflammatory properties of the virus.

Why are SSRIs effective in treating COVID? In patients with COVID, SSRIs may help limit the cytokine release process that is partly responsible for worsening the illness's inflammatory component.

Researchers at Yale University published initial evidence that two drugs used to treat attention deficit disorder can lessen or even eliminate brain fog. Guanfacine was approved by the Food and Drug Administration (FDA) for treating ADHD in 2009, but clinicians have also used it extensively off-label for other brain disorders, such as traumatic brain injury and PTSD. Arman Fesharaki-Zadeh, MD, PhD, assistant professor of psychiatry and neurology at Yale University, has been treating long COVID patients with a combination of guanfacine and N-acetylcysteine (NAC), an antioxidant also used for the treatment of traumatic brain injury. The combined therapy was successful in relieving brain fog for a small group of individuals. While larger, placebo-controlled clinical trials are needed to establish these drugs as a bona fide treatment for post-COVID neurocognitive deficits, patients can obtain them now if their doctors wish to prescribe them.

Exercise. According to Dr. Lisa Sanders at Yale Medical School, physical activity might be the key to lessening some acute and lasting symptoms of COVID-19, particularly psychological and neurological symptoms. She cites a study in Hungary where investigators found that young women who suffered from long COVID-19 symptoms and exercised fared better than those who did not.

In addition, those who did the most exercise, at least two and a half hours per week, reported fewer post-COVID-19 symptoms than their nonexercising counterparts. The researchers believe the difference is due to exercise's known benefits, including boosting the immune system and improving cardiovascular fitness.

Nutrition. A study in *Nutrients* suggests that nutrition could play a key role in managing long COVID-19 and other infections. One of the side effects of prolonged infection is a loss of muscle mass. This is particularly true in older individuals and those who were prescribed steroids to reduce the disease-related inflammation. They recommend a diet high in protein with 15 to 30 grams per meal and possible creatinine supplementation, which helps build muscle mass and protects your brain. Some patients with long-term symptoms have dysregulation in their gut environment, mainly if antibiotics are prescribed. Their recommendations are for a balanced diet, like the Mediterranean diet, that supports the growth of healthy bacteria.

Vitamin C is an antioxidant with immune-modulating properties.

One study involving 720 patients found that two-thirds of those receiving vitamin C supplementation experienced marked reductions in fatigue scores and improvements in concentration, sleep hygiene, and depression compared to those who did not.

A study is currently underway to investigate the possible benefits of probiotic supplementation in patients with long COVID symptoms. Some researchers believe that COVID's disruption of the natural gut biome contributes to long-haul symptoms. We know the gut and brain are intimately connected, so the theory makes sense. Probiotics have few, if any, side effects and are available over the counter, so trying this option has little risk.

Dhyana. Calming practices such as mindfulness training and meditation have been proven helpful in many inflammatory disorders, both infectious and autoimmune. Brain retraining can calm your nervous system and reduce inflammation, as well as improve brain fog. You can start with five to ten minutes per day using meditation apps like Calm or Headspace or through other free content online.

Sleep. Sleep is critical for good overall health and is especially important when recovering from an infectious disease. Long COVID is believed to be due to a prolonged and protracted low-grade inflammatory process. Therefore, it has been hypothesized that a pharmacological agent with antioxidative effects may be beneficial in treating the syndrome. Melatonin is a drug that activates Nrf2, a protein believed to increase the formation of antioxidants on a cellular level. In addition, melatonin has beneficial effects on sleep disturbances.

Patients with post-Lyme syndrome often report sleep disturbances. According to a study by Johns Hopkins University School of Medicine, researchers found that PTLDS participants reported significantly worse overall sleep and sleep disturbance scores, and worse fatigue, functional impact, and more cognitive-affective depressive symptoms compared to even poor-sleeping controls. Some patients suffering from chronic pain that is affecting their sleep gain benefit from a medication called gabapentin taken at bedtime. Others prefer the older tricyclic antidepressants that can help with insomnia as well as chronic pain.

Lemon balm and melatonin are nonpharmacologic options generally considered safe. Other supplements that I have recommended are evening primrose and valerian, which are similar to Valium but are not medications and are not habit-forming.

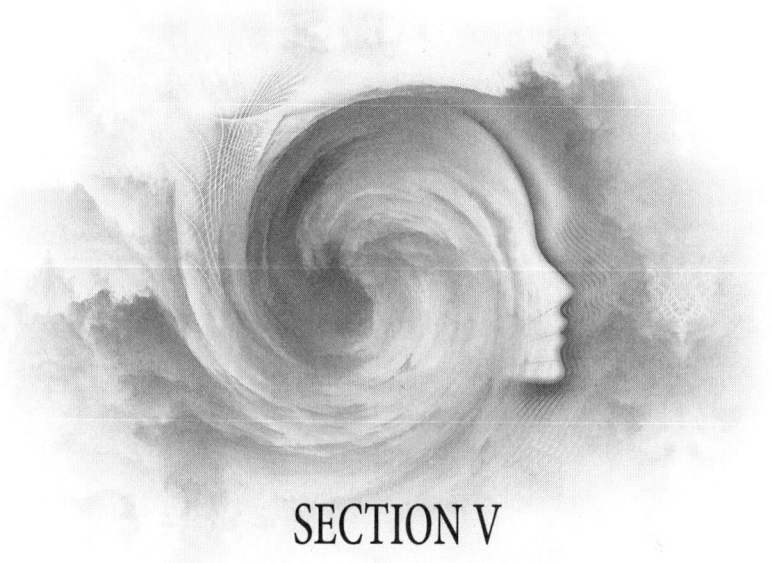

SECTION V

• • •

YOUR BRAIN ON FIRE

CHAPTER 10

INFLAMMATION AND BRAIN FUNCTION

*With sixty staring me in the face,
I have developed inflammation
of the sentence structure and
definite hardening of
the paragraphs.*
—JAMES THURBER

How many times have you cut yourself by accident? Did you ever wonder how the wound heals? Perhaps you needed surgery, and during your recovery, did you notice the changing color and texture of your incision site? Do you believe it is a bad sign when you contract an infection and raise a fever? Each of these scenarios describes your body's response to an assault, which could be infectious, intentional trauma such as an operation, or an accidental injury. The phenomenon that explains how our bodies react when it believes it is under attack is called "inflammation."

Our understanding of inflammation dates to the first century, when Roman medical writer Aulus Cornelius Celsus described the four cardinal features of inflammation: heat, swelling, pain, and redness. Later in the century, the Greek medical researcher Galen added a fifth feature: loss of function.

An inflammatory response occurs when bacteria, trauma, toxins, heat, or other factors injure your tissues. During this process, white blood cells rush to the injured area to fight infection, followed by blood-borne cells called *monocytes*. The monocytes reside inside the tissue, and cells called *macrophages* release compounds called *cytokines*, which signal other inflammatory proteins. Soon, immune cells flood the site, destroying foreign invaders and damaged tissue. Once the pathogens are eradicated, the inflammatory process recedes and makes way for healing.

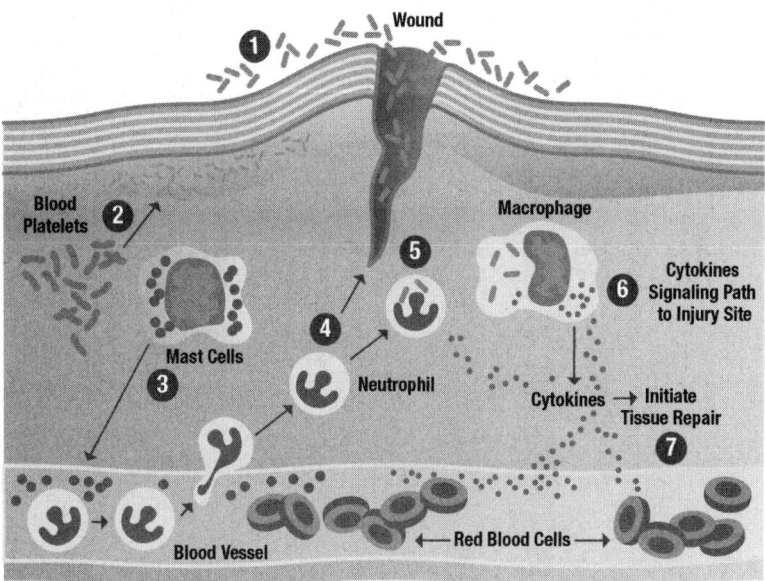

1. Bacteria and other pathogens enter wound.
2. Platelets from blood release blood-clotting proteins at wound site.
3. Mast cells secrete factors that mediate vasodilation and vascular constriction. Delivery of blood, plasma, and cells to injured area increases.
4. Neutrophils secrete factors that kill and degrade pathogens.
5. Neutrophils and macrophages remove pathogens by phagocytosis.
6. Macrophages secrete hormones called cytokines that attract immune system cells to the site and activate cells involved in tissue repair.
7. Inflammatory response continues until the foreign material is eliminated and the wound is repaired.

Fig. 10.1 The Inflammatory Response

Inflammation is our body's defense mechanism against phenomena it recognizes as foreign. However, as with any complicated defense system, an error can occur. When that happens, your immune system incorrectly identifies a part of your body as an invader and inappropriately launches an attack. The same physiological process that reddens your skin and raises a welt after an insect bite can misfire and lead to a host of ailments, ranging from cancer and depression to diabetes and severe cases of COVID-19.

Inflammation usually helps our bodies fight bacteria, viruses, and other toxins. However, if the immune response continues unchecked after the threat has passed, it can damage healthy tissue.

The Health Effects of Chronic Inflammation

According to an article published by the National Library of Medicine, chronic inflammatory diseases are the most significant cause of death worldwide. In 2000, nearly 125 million Americans were living with chronic conditions, and 21 percent had more than one. In the scientific community, several theories explain why chronic inflammation occurs:

- A failure of your immune system to completely eliminate infections resistant to your natural defenses, so they remain in your tissues for extended periods.
- Exposure to a low level of an irritant or a foreign material that cannot be eliminated from your body. This could include industrial chemicals for those working in environments where they are regularly exposed to low-level toxins.
- The development of an autoimmune disorder that attacks the body's cells and creates a vicious cycle of inflammation.
- The phenomenon of oxidative stress. Oxidative stress is an imbalance between two different types of molecules in your body: free radicals and antioxidants. Specifically, it means there are too many free radicals and not enough antioxidants. As a result, the excess free radicals start to harm your body's cells and tissues.
- A genetic defect in the cells that regulate inflammation causes a persistent infection to develop.

Several factors may put you at risk for developing chronic inflammation. Many studies report that obesity may be a contributor to chronic disease by inducing inflammation. Fat tissues in your body secrete inflammatory substances. Evidence shows that an individual's body mass index (BMI) is proportional to the number of inflammatory proteins produced. Smoking cigarettes is an additional risk factor. Aside from contributing to cancer and chronic lung disease, the contents of cigarette smoke lower your body's production of anti-inflammatory molecules. We all know that adequate sleep is essential for good overall health. Research now documents that physical and psychological stress are associated with the release of inflammatory proteins. Stress is a negative factor in the production of restorative sleep, and people with sleep disorders have higher levels of chronic inflammation.

Every day, our bodies carry out complex processes that we are unaware of, but that are astonishing and contribute to our overall health. For instance, did you know that your body has a built-in power-washing system to remove toxins and free radicals from your central nervous system? In 2012, scientists discovered that the glymphatic system does just that. The key here is that the glymphatic system is highly active during sleep and is disengaged during wakefulness. So, if you do not sleep well, you rob your body of the ability to clear out the leftovers of your day, causing the potential buildup of waste products linked to degenerative brain disorders.

An additional risk factor for chronic inflammation is age. The older we get, the higher our levels of inflammatory molecules. This may be related to age-associated factors such as increased fat tissue or declining levels of sex hormones. Research studies report that testosterone and estrogen can suppress the presence of inflammatory markers.

What Is Inflammaging?

As we age, our immune system may struggle to mount the necessary response to attack invading pathogens and limit collateral damage to our tissues. This phenomenon is known as *immunosenescence*. As we grow older, our immune system deteriorates, and the reaction to a pathogen may shift from a robust response to a more subdued one, resulting in unresolved inflammation. This kind of inflammation is referred to as *inflammaging*—a chronic, persistent inflammatory response that fails to combat pathogens but accumulates over time, damaging tissues. As mentioned earlier, this condition increases our risk for chronic inflammation and associated diseases, including many of the autoimmune disorders illustrated below.

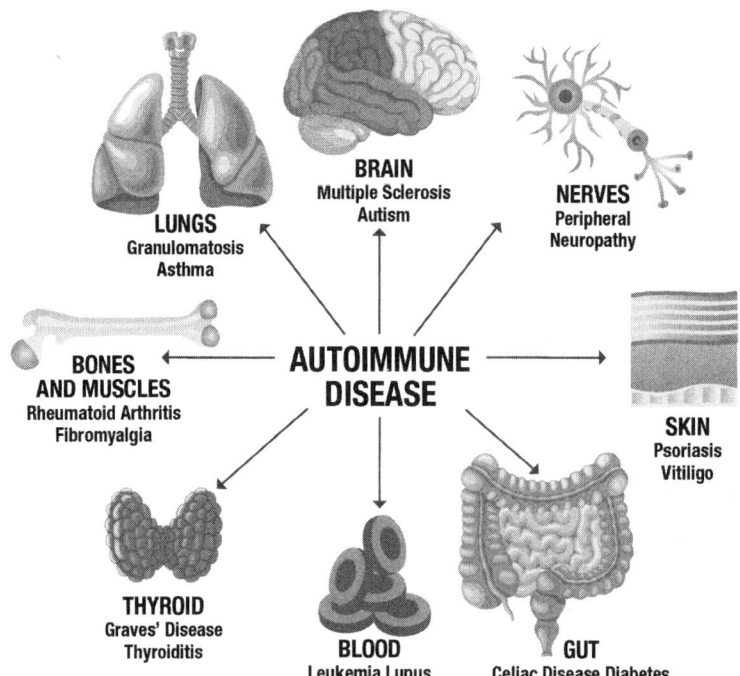

Fig. 10.2 Autoimmune Disorders Can Target Various Organ Systems

The Hygiene Hypothesis

What helps to explain the increased global prevalence of autoimmune disorders? The hygiene hypothesis suggests that the increased incidence of allergic and autoimmune disorders in the last century is linked to tremendous changes in sanitation standards and practices in developing countries during the Industrial Revolution. On face value, this appears counterintuitive. While infectious agents are potentially responsible for many diseases, the theory emerged that these agents could, in some cases, have a favorable effect on noninfectious and sometimes severe illnesses.

Public health measures taken by Western countries after the Industrial Revolution limited the spread of infections. These measures included the creation of a clean water supply, pasteurization and sterilization of milk and other food products, refrigeration of perishable products, vaccination against common childhood infections, and the widespread use of antibiotics. In countries where good health standards do not exist, people are chronically infected by various pathogens, but the prevalence of allergic diseases remains low. Interestingly, several countries that have eradicated common infections are now seeing the emergence of allergic and autoimmune diseases. In fact, the geographical distribution of allergic and autoimmune diseases mirrors the geographical distribution of various infectious diseases.

The hygiene hypothesis proposes that childhood exposure to germs and certain infections helps develop our immune system. In this theory, early exposure to germs teaches our immune system not to overreact. In support of this, children growing up in rural areas, around animals, and in larger families are less likely to develop asthma than children without this exposure.

In 1989, researcher D. P. Strachan reported that hay fever and allergic dermatitis are less frequent in families with many children than in families with only one or two children. In 2000, he proposed his theory that the increase in allergic diseases observed in the three or four preceding decades could be attributed to the decrease in some common infectious diseases. In the early 2000s, the hygiene hypothesis was extended to include autoimmune diseases based on data obtained in experimental models showing that infections, particularly parasitic infections, could prevent the occurrence of autoimmunity.

Researchers suggest that exposure to certain germs before birth may play an essential role in developing a baby's immune system and gut microbiome. A 2022 study published in *Digestive Diseases* reported a much higher amount of healthy gut bacteria in children exposed to household pets while still in utero. Exposure to dogs, particularly after birth and during the ages of five to fifteen, was linked with a healthy gut and immune response. This is unsurprising since we have already learned that your gut is heavily involved in your immune system.

The Link Between Chronic Inflammation and Psychiatric Disorders

Cytokine-induced sickness behavior is a syndrome characterized by decreased activity, depression, and loss of energy due to increased circulating levels of cytokines, the pro-inflammatory proteins we explored earlier. These proteins are released during the process of inflammation. In research studies, this syndrome has been proposed as a model for the role the immune system plays in depression. Recent evidence indicates that chronic inflammation is linked to the development of psychiatric disorders. For example, increased levels of inflammatory proteins have been found in patients with disorders such as schizophrenia and depression.

In animal models, stress was linked to an increase in an inflammatory protein believed to contribute to the development of depression. Inhibition of this protein prevented the development of depression in these animals. In human studies, blood levels of an inflammatory protein were found in depressed patients compared to healthy volunteers. In one Japanese study, researchers found elevated levels of inflammatory markers in the spinal fluid of depressed patients compared to the control group.

Interferon-based therapies work by activating an antiviral immune response and are used to treat hepatitis C. In one study, almost 20 percent of the patients receiving this therapy developed psychiatric side effects, primarily depression. However, the symptoms resolved upon discontinuation of treatment. Similar results have been found in patients receiving antiviral therapies for melanoma, a serious skin cancer. Interestingly, these symptoms responded well to antidepressant medication.

The role of inflammation in depression and fatigue led researchers to examine how inflammation in our peripheral nervous system affects our central nervous system. They found that during inflammation, changes occur in the blood-brain barrier. This barrier becomes more porous during inflammation, allowing the entry of pro-inflammatory proteins. This has been proposed as a theory for the development of long COVID-19, which is associated with psychiatric symptoms, including depression. In animal models, this process was reversed using anti-inflammatory drugs.

Over 9,000 studies have investigated the role of the immune system in depression, particularly the role of inflammation. As a result of this data, researchers are investigating whether anti-inflammatory drugs can be used successfully, either alone or in conjunction with traditional antidepressants, to improve outcomes in patients with treatment-resistant depression. One of these drugs, Celecoxib, is an inhibitor of an enzyme called COX-2 that is involved in inflammation. It has been the most extensively studied NSAID (nonsteroidal anti-inflammatory drug) for depression. Multiple small-scale randomized controlled trials found that when added to standard antidepressant treatment (such as fluoxetine, sertraline, or reboxetine), celecoxib (typically at a dose of 400 mg/day for six weeks) led to significantly greater improvements in depressive symptoms, higher response rates, and better remission rates compared to antidepressants alone with a placebo.

A recent study published in *Nature* reported the findings of research that looked at the effect of high levels of inflammation on the development of low motivation. The study enrolled forty-two subjects who were diagnosed with depression and also exhibited high levels of inflammation as measured by a blood test called C-reactive protein. They were randomly divided into two groups. One group of subjects received a single dose of an anti-inflammatory medication used to treat arthritis. The other group received a placebo. The researchers studied the subjects for two weeks, during which they were asked to perform various tasks and complete questionnaires designed to measure motivation levels. The results showed that the group that received the anti-inflammatory drug had an increased willingness to engage in tasks associated with rewards.

Depression is a debilitating mental health disorder that affects almost 300 million people worldwide and is a leading cause of disability and premature death. The World Health Organization considers depression to be a significant cause of global disease burden and predicts it will be a leading contributor by 2030. Almost one-third of patients with major depression have treatment-resistant disease. This is defined as a lack of response to adequate antidepressant trials and can be due to many factors, including noncompliance, coexisting substance abuse, and ongoing physical illness. As more research explores the role of inflammation in the development of depression, additional options for treating resistant disease will emerge. Inflammation plays a potential role in the etiology of depression, and anti-inflammatory intervention may represent a novel way of developing more personalized treatment regimens for some patients.

Why do some people develop autoimmune disorders while others do not? Autoimmune disorders do run in families, but this is not always the case. The hygiene theory of autoimmunity is not proven but is an interesting idea that has some support in the scientific community. Other theories have been proposed, but the bottom line is that we still do not know why some individuals have an immune system that misreads their body's cues and attacks its own cells.

In the context of medically unexplained symptoms, autoimmune disorders often present in unusual ways, so it is not uncommon for me to diagnose an autoimmune disorder in a new patient who arrives in my waiting room after seeing multiple specialists who cannot determine a diagnosis. Sarah is one example.

Sarah was a tall, athletic young woman who attended a local university. She was an excellent student with high expectations to obtain exceptional grades. She was also on a varsity athletic team that required her to wake early, often before sunrise, to train for two hours before classes started. She was taking a full course load and hoped to attend law school after graduation.

Along with the rigors of her schedule, Sarah was also experiencing a great deal of stress elsewhere in her life. She hoped to study abroad the following semester but had yet to receive a definite placement. Her athletic coach was demanding and could be harsh with Sarah and her team members if they failed to meet his high expectations. Her home life was difficult as well. Her parents were in a long-term, contentious relationship, and one of her two brothers had just entered rehab for drug addiction. Sarah was the "golden child" in the family, having performed well in high school, abstained from drugs and alcohol, and worked part-time after school. Despite this, she often felt neglected by her parents, who were both professionals and who spent a great deal of time worrying about her brother's substance abuse problems.

Sarah developed an eating disorder in high school and it was still active when I started working with her. With the help of an excellent therapist, her eating disorder was currently under control. The medication I prescribed when she started college had been keeping her depression and anxiety under control, until now.

When Sarah arrived in my office, she did not look well. Although she denied the return of her eating disorder, she looked thin and pale. She told me she was not sleeping well and always felt tired.

"Not only am I always tired, but my joints also ache, and I have this weird redness in my hands and feet," she said.

I wondered if some of her symptoms could be due to a re-emergence of her past depression that had been in remission for months. Sleep and appetite issues are common in mood disorders, as are fatigue and memory loss. However, she described additional symptoms.

"This is different than when I was depressed," she said. "I feel like my brain is stuck in a cloud, and it is just foggy."

I asked her to remove her shoes so I could see her feet to see if they were as red as her hands were. They looked fine to me.

"Wait," she said. "I took pictures of them when they were red." She showed me the photo on her phone, which clearly showed her bright red feet.

Honestly, I had never seen anything quite like this, but I knew it was not the result of depression. The constellation of brain fog, redness, achiness, sleep problems, and appetite issues made me think an autoimmune disorder might be causing her symptoms. I referred Sarah to a local rheumatologist and waited to hear back after her first appointment.

Weeks later, Sarah called to tell me the symptoms I saw were due to a rare autoimmune disorder called *erythromelalgia*. The other interesting fact she reported was that the rheumatologist diagosed not one but three autoimmune disorders including Hashimoto's thyroiditis, myasthenia gravis, and fibromyalgia. The psychiatric symptoms she reported were most likely due to the inflammation in her body that was also affecting her brain.

How Does Stress Lead to Inflammation?

In the last two decades, researchers discovered that severe or prolonged (chronic) stress can cause an increased risk for physical and psychiatric disorders. This is called *stress-related disease*. As with most systems in our bodies, there is direct communication between your neuroendocrine system, a network of cells that produce and release hormones into your bloodstream in response to signals from your nervous system, and your immune system. Your neuroendocrine system maintains balance in your body processes such as reproduction, growth, metabolism, energy balance, and stress responsiveness. When you experience either multiple stressors or one significant stressor for prolonged periods, your neuroendocrine system can produce more substantial amounts of the stress hormone cortisol, which can, in turn, lead to inflammation. Long-term studies on stress report that up to 80 percent of patients with autoimmune disorders reported experiencing uncommon emotional stress occurring prior to being diagnosed.

Unfortunately, not only does stress cause disease, but the disease itself may cause significant stress, resulting in a vicious cycle that magnifies the problem. Stress by itself may also aggravate or cause pain. The regions of the brain responsible for emotional and physical pain reside close to each other, and both areas may be triggered simultaneously during stress, resulting in a mutually reinforcing cycle that leads to chronic pain.

According to a study published in the *Journal of the American Medical Association*, a diagnosis of stress-related disorder is significantly associated with an increased risk of autoimmune disease. Further, the same study reported that individuals who experienced extreme stress were more likely to have multiple autoimmune disorders, just like Sarah.

Why Are More Women Diagnosed with Autoimmune Disorders?

Women are more than four times more likely than men to be diagnosed with autoimmune disorders. Many explanations are proposed to account for this difference, including sex hormones, women's extra X chromosome, environmental factors, and differences in our gut environment. Understanding the mechanism for this difference is essential because autoimmune disorders are a leading cause of morbidity and mortality in young and middle-aged women. One theory postulates that the discrepancy is because women have higher circulating levels of antibodies than their male counterparts. The exception is men who have a condition called Klinefelter's syndrome. Men born with this condition have an extra copy of the X chromosome; they also have higher levels of antibodies. In addition, their prevalence of autoimmune disorders is equal to that of women.

Researchers at two major medical centers investigated this difference from an evolutionary perspective. They wondered why nature would preserve excess antibody production in women, particularly during their prime childbearing years. For example, women's antibody levels spike after giving birth. This is also the time that they are more likely to be diagnosed with autoimmune disorders. They believe the answer is related to infections. Infections are a leading cause of death for infants and adults. Even in the modern world, almost 70 percent of infant deaths are attributed to an infectious disease. So, from an evolutionary perspective, women having higher antibodies during their reproductive years means they are more likely to fight off infections, and if breastfed, their infants have the same advantage.

Women have two X chromosomes while men have an X and a Y chromosome. The X chromosome contains more genetic material than the Y and carries more immune-related genes. Because of this, the X chromosome has a greater probability of containing gene-related mutations.

A study at the University of California, Los Angeles (UCLA) discovered that a gene located on the X chromosome could explain why women are more prone to develop multiple sclerosis (MS) than men. The researchers found a gene called KDM6A that is more frequently expressed in women's immune cells. In an animal study modeling

MS-like disease, researchers found that female mice missing the KDM6A gene developed significantly less inflammation and sustained less spinal cord injury than normal mice.

A Stanford University study supports the theory that women's extra X chromosomes is the reason for their increased risk of autoimmune disorders. The study focused on a molecule called Xist, which is found on the X chromosome. This molecule is only transcribed into RNA proteins when two XX chromosomes are present. Its job is to shut down the extra X chromosome in a process called X-chromosome inactivation. The study's lead author, Howard Chang, found that Xist can occasionally form unusual RNA combinations that bind to other proteins, creating complexes capable of triggering a strong immune response.

To eliminate the sex difference, his group studied male mice genetically altered to contain an Xist protein who were bred to be susceptible to autoimmune disorders. Once the researchers chemically activated the Xist complex in those animals, they developed symptoms like human lupus, an autoimmune disorder. When the researchers stimulated the Xist molecule in male mice bred to be resistant to autoimmunity, they did not have the same result. This mirrors what is seen in humans: Women are more susceptible to autoimmune disorders, yet not all women develop them.

One of the most common signs of brain inflammation is brain fog—a feeling of slowed, fuzzy thinking. Other frequent symptoms include depression, anxiety, irritability, anger, memory problems, and fatigue.

Symptoms of autoimmune disorders are frequently mischaracterized as psychiatric illnesses. There is tremendous overlap in areas such as sleep, appetite, fatigue, and poor concentration. Some differences, however, delineate the two. It is unlikely for me to see a patient with rashes, joint pain, or problems regulating their internal temperature that can solely be attributed to a mood disorder. Medical providers need to understand the difference because it is sometimes a matter of life or death. Journalist Susannah Cahalan brought this to light in her book *Brain on Fire*. In it, she describes her firsthand experience of being misdiagnosed with bipolar disorder when, in fact, she had a form of encephalitis, inflammation of her brain.

CHAPTER 11

WHEN THE BODY ATTACKS ITSELF: THE MYSTERIES OF AUTOIMMUNE DISORDERS AND RELATED PHENOMENA

*I can be changed by what happens to me,
but I refuse to be reduced by it.*
—MAYA ANGELOU

Remember Allie from Chapter 9? I met her when she was on leave from an Ivy League college after she was diagnosed with mononucleosis, the "kissing disease" caused by the Epstein-Barr virus. Allie kept in touch with me during her remaining college years and graduated with honors. She had been doing so well that I was surprised by a phone call I received from Allie's worried mother two years after my last appointment with her daughter. This is a summary of our conversation:

"Thanks for taking my call, Dr. Trachman. Allie did so well after seeing you that I know she didn't schedule a follow-up appointment."

"That's okay," I said. I'm always glad to hear that my patients have done well. "What's going on now?"

"Well, Allie did graduate with honors. She worked hard, and you know how kids party at the end of their senior year? She wasn't sleeping much, was drinking alcohol with her friends, and going on senior trips, like to the lake and to breweries.

"After she graduated, she wanted to go on a cross-country road trip with some of her friends before starting her summer job and taking her required premed classes because late in her senior year, she decided she wanted to go to medical school. When she returned from her trip, she was clearly exhausted. She constantly complained about being tired, but my husband and I assumed it was because of the activity and excitement around graduation. Still, she wanted to go with us to our beach house for a long weekend before her job at the hospital started. It was a great weekend; the weather was perfect, but Allie got a bad sunburn.

"Even after sleeping for ten hours, she complained of being tired. One morning, she woke up early and called for me.

'Mom,' she said, 'my head hurts so bad I just can't move.'

"Dr. Trachman, I thought it was just a migraine, so I gave her some Tylenol, but it did nothing. I had some Percocet from a recent dental procedure and tried that. All it did was tire her, with no effect on the pain. Now I was getting worried. We could go to urgent care or drive home so that she could see one of our doctors, but Allie wanted to stay. She had invited some of her college friends to join us, and they were arriving the next day. I had to return home from work, and my husband had already left to care for our dogs. Her college friends are very reliable, and I felt she would be in good hands if I left. Allie said it was okay, so I did.

"While I was at work the following day, I received a call from one of her friends who told me Allie couldn't get out of bed and complained that her head was hurting. I asked them to drag her into the car and head home. Allie didn't have a regular doctor after having aged out of her pediatrician's practice, and my doctor had no appointments available for at least a week. I didn't think it could wait, so I would have to take her to the emergency room at one of our local hospitals.

"The girls arrived later in the day. Allie looked terrible. Her headache hadn't improved, and the sunburn on her face looked worse. I wondered if they could be related. I got her into my car and headed to the emergency room. Luckily, it was midday, so the ER wasn't busy. Allie was admitted, and the doctors took a history, then started to draw blood and ordered a CT of her head. She asked for some pain medication, as they started an IV then added morphine.

"When her blood test came back, the doctors looked worried. Her blood count was very low, so low that they were thinking about transfusing her. But first they wanted to consult a hematologist.

"Dr. Lee arrived a short time later, and after reviewing all of the reports and listening to the history, he said a transfusion could kill her. He believed she was experiencing a form of hemolytic anemia, when the body attacks and destroys its own blood cells. Dr. Lee believed a transfusion would only make that worse. He suggested a rheumatology consult because he believed she had an autoimmune disorder. In the meantime, he admitted her to the ICU for observation and started her on steroids to calm her immune reaction."

"My goodness, I am so sorry to hear this," I said. "It must be awful for all of you. What can I do to help?"

"Nothing right now. The rheumatologist was on vacation but will be in to see Allie tomorrow. I think she's safe in the hospital. We can only hope the steroids work and they find an answer. We'll reach out to you when she's discharged. I'm sure she'll want to see you. This has been quite an ordeal. She's devastated that she can't start her job. Her premed classes are supposed to begin next month."

After our conversation ended, I pulled out Allie's old chart. I reminded myself that she had a bout of Epstein-Barr virus when I last saw her. I knew that EBV was sometimes linked to autoimmune disorders that develop later in life. Allie fit the profile, both in sex and age, as autoimmune disorders occur most frequently in females of reproductive age.

I received another phone call from Allie's mother about a week later. Allie was discharged from the hospital and was recovering at home. The rheumatologist saw her and believed this was her first bout with lupus. She was taking high doses of oral steroids to reduce her symptoms. They were going to follow her blood work, and she planned to make an appointment to see me after she felt better.

A History of the Lupus Diagnosis

In 1851, physicians introduced the name lupus erythematosus for a disease typically identified by a red facial rash that looks like a wolf's bite. Lupus is a chronic autoimmune disease where the immune system mistakenly attacks the body's own healthy tissues and organs, causing widespread inflammation and damage, often affecting joints, skin, kidneys, heart, lungs, and brain, with symptoms varying from mild to severe, including fatigue, fever, and sometimes a butterfly-shaped facial rash. Lupus is a spectrum disorder. By that, I mean it can affect the entire body and multiple organ systems. This is referred to as *systemic lupus erythematosus* (SLE), which is the most common form present in 70 percent of people.

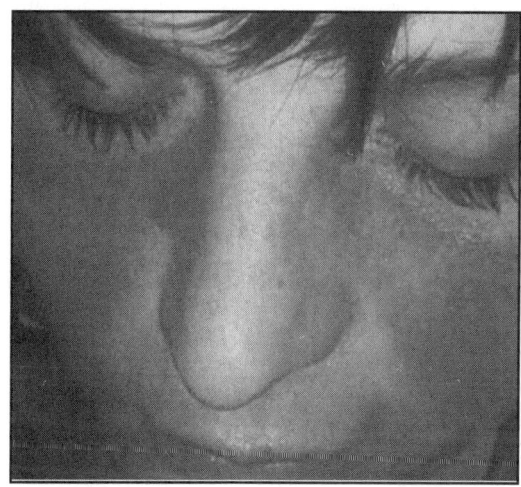

Fig. 11.1 Young Woman with a Classic Lupus Rash

However, some forms of lupus are limited to only one body system. For example, cutaneous lupus is limited to the skin, although it may eventually progress to SLE in some patients. Lupus-like symptoms can even occur as the result of taking prescribed medications such as Isoniazid, used to treat tuberculosis; hydralazine, used to treat high blood pressure; and even minocycline, an antibiotic prescribed for acne. This is called drug-induced lupus. It has many of the same symptoms as SLE but rarely affects major organ systems and usually disappears within six months. The remainder of this chapter is devoted to the neuropsychiatric symptoms of lupus, the type of disorder I commonly see.

What Are the Neuropsychiatric Symptoms Caused by Lupus?

Neuropsychiatric lupus (NPSLE) refers to the neurological and psychiatric results of SLE. NPSLE can be challenging for physicians to manage. The prevalence of NPSLE in patients with SLE is 30 to 40 percent, and 50 to 60 percent of these patients develop NPSLE within one year of the SLE onset. The different types of neuropsychiatric manifestations of SLE are shown below.

Neuropsychiatric Manifestations in Systemic Lupus Erythematosus

	Central Nervous System (CNS)	**Peripheral Nervous System (PNS)**
Diffuse manifestations	Acute confusional state Anxiety disorder Cognitive dysfunction Mood disorders Psychosis	
Focal manifestations	Aseptic meningitis Cerebrovascular disease Demyelinating syndrome Headache Movement disorder Myelopathy Seizures	Guillain-Barré syndrome Autonomic disorder Mononeuropathy, single/ multiplex Myasthenia gravis Neuropathy, cranial Plexopathy Polyneuropathy

Table. 11.1 Manifestations of Central and Peripheral Nervous System Disorders

The diffuse symptoms affect the entire body while the focal manifestations are specific to one location. For example, seizures are specific to the brain, and myelopathy refers to muscle pain and weakness. It's important to understand that not everyone diagnosed with SLE will experience the full range of symptoms. Some of the common neuropsychiatric symptoms of lupus include confusion, difficulty concentrating, seizures, headaches, and stroke.

CNS lupus can also cause some rare but serious problems, including psychosis (a disturbance in thought and perception of reality) and myelitis (inflammation of the spinal cord).

Lupus can cause nerve damage due to inflammation of the nerves themselves or their surrounding tissue. This is called *peripheral neuropathy*. The main symptoms are numbness, tingling, and decreased mobility.

Other symptoms include loss of vision, facial pain, tinnitus, hearing changes, and dizziness. Many people with lupus have other nervous system problems, like headaches, depression, and anxiety. One of the most common and bothersome symptoms is lupus fog.

What Is Lupus Fog?

Lupus fog is a general term for the cognitive impairments that often appear with lupus, including concentration and memory problems, confusion, and difficulty with verbal or written expression. These problems frequently worsen during disease flares. The exact cause of lupus fog is not fully understood. Researchers believe that, in some cases, lupus can directly damage brain cells, leading to cognitive problems. However, in most cases, other factors play a role, including fatigue, stress, and depression. Lupus fog is sometimes worse in people who also have fibromyalgia, a long-term condition that causes pain in muscles and soft tissues. Sometimes, the fog can be attributed to the medications prescribed to patients during a lupus flare.

Medications like prednisone work by suppressing your immune system, which is how they improve symptoms. However, they are not innocuous drugs. The side effects of prednisone can include sleep problems, overeating, irritability, mood swings, extreme fatigue, and sometimes even manic-like symptoms if they are prescribed at high doses. As a third-year resident, I was called to see a young woman admitted for a lupus flare. The nurses were concerned that she was irritable, combative, and appeared to be responding to invisible stimuli. She was speaking rapidly, but her language was unintelligible. After reviewing her chart, I noted that her attending physician raised her steroid dose the day before. He was concerned that her disease was causing kidney damage. Sometimes, high doses of steroids can cause this type of mental confusion. The only way to know for sure is to lower the steroid dose. If the mental confusion improves, it was caused by the steroids. If they get worse, the disease itself is causing the problem. This is known as *lupus encephalitis*, when the inflammation from the disease causes the brain to malfunction.

Back to Allie...

"Hi, Allie," I said as she entered my office about a month after her mother first called me.

"Hi, Dr. Trachman. It's been quite a ride since I last saw you. A lot has happened."

"Please fill me in," I said as she sat on my couch.

"It was scary. I didn't know what had happened to me. One minute, I was graduating from college, having fun with my friends, partying to celebrate being done. Then suddenly, I couldn't move. It was like a heavy stone. I couldn't get out of bed; my head was pounding, and nothing made it better, not even morphine, which only made me more tired and gave me weird nightmares. Being in the ICU was the worst; they told me I could have died. I'm so young and healthy. How could I have ended up in this situation?"

"Allie, you didn't do anything wrong. There were a lot of stressors in your life. Even good things can be stressful. Although autoimmune disorders are prevalent in young women, it doesn't mean you can't have a normal life. You will have to take precautions," I told her.

"I'm feeling pretty anxious and depressed right now, to be honest. I'm not sure if it's the medication I'm taking or just the fact that I have to adjust to having a chronic illness at such a young age. I wanted to attend medical school, but now I'm not sure that I can."

"Allie," I began, "there's nothing unusual about having symptoms after learning about a consequential diagnosis. I'm sure the steroids had something to do with the onset of the depression and anxiety. They are often linked. There is no reason you cannot fulfill your dream of attending medical school because you have an autoimmune disorder. You will have to learn to take precautions so that you don't have additional flares when things get really stressful. Let's talk about a treatment plan for you for the next few months," I suggested.

Allie's mother had a good response to an antidepressant called Cymbalta. Often, if a patient has a first-degree relative who has done well on a medication, it is a good idea to start with the same one.

I started Allie on a low dose of Cymbalta. We discussed her plans for taking some time off to recover from her lupus flare. The rheumatologist she was seeing suggested starting her on a medication called Plaquenil to prevent a recurrence of her symptoms. We discussed ensuring that she practiced good sleep hygiene, ate healthy foods (including those with anti-inflammatory properties), limited her alcohol consumption, and got regular exercise.

I planned to see her again in a month and then regularly while she was home over the summer. She hoped to begin her premed classes at a local university in the fall.

What Is an Anti-Inflammatory Diet?

The medical profession is learning that one of the best ways to reduce inflammation lies not in the medicine cabinet but in the refrigerator. Aim for an overall healthy diet, and if you're looking for an eating plan that closely follows the tenets of anti-inflammatory eating, consider the Mediterranean diet, which is high in fruits, vegetables, nuts, whole grains, fish, and healthy oils.

In addition to lowering inflammation, eating more natural, whole, minimally processed foods can have noticeable effects on your physical and emotional health. A healthy diet is beneficial for reducing the risk of chronic diseases and improving your mood and overall quality of life.

Specific Recommendations for Dealing with Lupus Fog Symptoms

- **Keep a log.** Lighten the load on your memory by keeping written notes and lists.
- **Keep an organizer.** Daily planners are invaluable. Jotting down all your tasks and activities in one place will help you stay organized.
- **Prioritize tasks.** You do not have to do everything at once. Decide on two or three tasks for the day and do your best to complete them. You can build on success this way.
- **Exercise your mind.** Crossword puzzles, word searches and jumbles, and Sudoku are great, fun ways to stretch your brain and keep your memory sharp.

CHAPTER 12

WHEN YOU'RE RUNNING ON EMPTY: CHRONIC FATIGUE SYNDROME

*If I say, "I have chronic fatigue syndrome,"
I'm likely to be discredited as a witness to my own condition.
I've had doctors tell me there's no such thing as chronic fatigue
syndrome. One doctor said, "Just drink some coffee."*
—TONI BERNHARD, author

Jessica was the daughter of two physicians and employed in a high-level position at a government agency. Married with two children, she was knowledgeable and spent a good deal of time learning about medical conditions from her father, an internist, and from Dr. Google—well, you know who he is and might be acquainted with him yourself. Unlike many of my new patients, she wasn't wondering what was wrong with her. She was certain that she knew the problem.

"I think I know what is wrong with me," Jessica said as she made herself comfortable on my couch.

"What's that?" I asked, wondering what she had concluded.

"I had to go into the office for the past month when they put in new carpet and painted the walls. I'm sure I was exposed to toxic fumes."

"What convinced you?" I asked.

"Well, I have a very sensitive system, and any kind of mold, fumes, or heavy perfume makes my body react in strange ways."

Jessica described a burning sensation running down her legs and back. She had daily headaches and was frequently fatigued. When she came home from work, she would nap, get up for dinner, and then go back to bed.

She told me about her family members and their dynamics. For the most part, they were high achievers. Her father, as mentioned, was an internist; her mother was a pediatrician; and her sister was a marketing executive. She also had a brother who did not fit the mold. She described him as an overweight, unmarried man who never truly found himself. Growing up, Jessica was her parents' favorite. She excelled academically and was a talented musician. In high school, she auditioned for and was invited to play in the state band—a major accomplishment. She did not excel athletically, preferring to read in her room.

Jessica's father was a perfectionist who demanded the same from his wife and children. Unfortunately, it was often difficult to meet his standards. As a result, he could become verbally and sometimes physically abusive, including using his belt as punishment. Jessica told me, "You never knew which father would show up after work: the nice daddy or the one who yelled. I knew he would be proud if

I did well in school or band. But if I dared to get a B grade, things would not go well for me."

Jessica told me that she developed an eating disorder when she was in law school. When stressed, she engaged in bingeing and purging of food as a way of maintaining a low body weight and also as a means of feeling in control. Fortunately, this was not active when she came to see me.

"I would like to know what is going on with me," she said. "I've seen my primary care doctor, who sent me to an infectious disease doctor, but my blood work returned normal. I don't think a tick bit me, but I did consider Lyme disease."

In addition to the reported physical symptoms, Jessica told me she lost interest in things that used to give her pleasure: gardening, cooking, and playing tennis. Some of these activities were limited due to her persistent low energy levels. However, she also described feeling sad most days and crying, which was unusual for her. She was anxious much of the time and was more irritable with her children. I considered the possibility that she might have chronic fatigue syndrome.

What Is Chronic Fatigue Syndrome?

Chronic fatigue syndrome (CFS) is a disabling long-term condition characterized by medically unexplained, persistent fatigue that is unimproved by rest and made worse by physical or mental activity. This fatigue is accompanied by other debilitating symptoms such as post-exertional malaise, confusion or slow thinking, muscle pain, joint pain, sleep disturbances, and hypersensitivity to incoming stimuli (like Jessica's hypersensitivity to smells). This describes many disorders such as those you've already read about. But CFS, as we will learn, is different.

Unlike lupus, objective tests or consistent biomarkers for CFS are not currently available. Consistent explanations for the physical manifestations sometimes remain elusive. It is no wonder, then, that patients who experience this disorder fall into the realm of "medically unexplained symptoms" and are sometimes not taken seriously by medical providers. Here are some things we do know:

- Approximately three-quarters of patients are female. Despite good intentions, gender bias persists in health care. A survey conducted in early 2019 found that more than half of women, compared with a third of men, believe gender discrimination in patient care is a serious problem. One in five women says that a healthcare provider has ignored or dismissed their symptoms, and 17 percent say they feel they have been treated differently because of their gender.
- Patients with CFS often experience chronic pain.
- Sufferers are typically in their forties at the first onset.
- Symptom severity varies both between patients and over time.
- Adults with CFS frequently experience depression and/or anxiety.
- In research studies, the maladaptive coping style known as perfectionism is linked to people who are eventually diagnosed with CFS.
- The onset of the disorder often follows a viral infection, such as COVID-19. Dr. Anthony Fauci said, "It's extraordinary how many people have a postviral syndrome that's very strikingly similar to myalgic encephalomyelitis/chronic fatigue syndrome."
- CFS impacts multiple organ systems, and the symptoms vary from patient to patient. Although many of the symptoms of

CFS overlap with those of other diseases, one feature that sets it apart is worsening of symptoms in response to relatively minor physical, cognitive, or emotional exertion. This is known as *postexertional malaise*.

This disorder frequently falls into the realm of psychiatry because, compared with the general population, patients with CFS have a higher risk of suicide. Suicidal thoughts may arise from the adverse effects on jobs and everyday activities, leading to feelings of inadequacy and diminished self-worth. Another important risk factor for suicide is chronic pain. Compounding this risk is the fact that CFS can be difficult to diagnose correctly, and patients with CFS may suffer from these symptoms for years.

Although the exact cause of CFS remains unknown, like most illnesses, recent research points to a multifactorial etiology. Some researchers propose that stressful or traumatic incidents in genetically vulnerable people may be the causative factor. These stressors can include infection, emotional stress, or significant life events.

More than 80 percent of patients diagnosed with CFS report that their symptoms began after an infection. Because CFS often appears after infection, some researchers believe the infection leads to an abnormal ongoing immune response characterized by excessive activity of inflammatory proteins, as we learned about in the previous section. A study published in *Nature Communications* looked at people who developed chronic fatigue syndrome after an infection and compared them with a healthy control group. All the participants spent a week at the National Institutes of Health and received daily testing. Those with CFS had been healthy before becoming ill with what seemed to them like a simple flu. They reported sore throat, coughing, aching muscles, and poor energy. However, unlike their past experiences with flu-like illnesses, they did not recover this time. For years, they experienced debilitating fatigue, difficulty thinking, and a flare of symptoms after exerting themselves physically or mentally. Some were so debilitated that they were bedridden or homebound. The results of the study were fascinating. The researchers found that the group experiencing CFS symptoms had long-standing immune system activation with increased circulating inflammatory proteins.

There is some evidence that the gut-brain connection is involved in the development of CFS. *Gut dysbiosis*, or an imbalance of the good and bad bacteria in your gut environment, can lead to increased permeability in the gut wall. Once this happens, harmful bacteria can leak out and travel through your bloodstream to distant organs. In support of this theory, researchers found that patients with CFS often have increased levels of harmful bacteria residing in their gut.

In 1969, the World Health Organization classified CFS as a neurological disorder. Aside from chronic fatigue syndrome, it is also known as *myalgic encephalomyelitis*. In everyday terms, this means people may experience muscle pain and inflammation in the brain and spinal cord. Brain scans often reveal this inflammation, which helps explain why affected individuals sometimes struggle with thinking, memory, and information processing.

The NIH study noted not only overactivation of participants' immune systems but also notable changes in their brain imaging. For example, the affected group had dysfunction in the area of their brain linked to fatigue. This area, the right temporal lobe, is typically related to motivation. In the affected subjects, their right temporal lobe was only mildly responsive, which usually looks activated on scans when people exert themselves. In addition, the cerebrospinal fluid (the fluid that bathes our brains and spinal cords) showed multiple differences in affected individuals versus the control group. These results point to objective brain changes in those experiencing chronic fatigue.

In addition to biological differences, research studies demonstrate that certain personality traits are linked to the development of CFS. Perfectionism is a tendency to set excessively high standards for yourself and others. In general, perfectionism is seen as a negative trait, but research shows both adaptive and maladaptive types of perfectionism. Adaptive perfectionism is seen in persistent and conscientious people in the face of adversity. Healthy perfectionism usually goes along with goal-directed behavior and good organizational skills. Examples of people with this type of perfectionism include elite athletes, entrepreneurs who create start-ups, doctors, or lawyers. These pursuits require perseverance, organizational skills, and a healthy drive in the face of difficult obstacles.

In contrast, maladaptive perfectionism is characterized by excessive preoccupation with past mistakes, fears about making new mistakes, doubts about whether you are doing something correctly, and being extremely concerned about the high expectations of others, such as parents or employers. A central feature of maladaptive perfectionism is an excessive preoccupation with being in control. It is perfectionism extreme enough to rule your life and cause severe anxiety. This type of perfectionism is linked to multiple medical conditions. If you recall, in a previous chapter, maladaptive perfectionism is a risk factor for cardiovascular disease.

CFS is associated with high rates of depression, and research increasingly indicates that both conditions overlap with respect to biological and psychological factors. For example, one study found that maladaptive perfectionism was positively related to the severity of fatigue and depression in a group of two hundred subjects with CFS. A 2021 research study examined the link between maladaptive perfectionism, depression, anxiety, and chronic fatigue syndrome. The researchers found that maladaptive perfectionism is consistently associated with depression in patients with CFS. The researchers proposed that maladaptive perfectionism, exceptionally high levels of self-criticism, and self-doubt may play an essential role in the development and propagation of CFS symptoms as a result of underlying depression.

Jessica's family had very high expectations for her. Her father was particularly demanding and likely suffered from maladaptive perfectionism. He clearly instilled the same in his daughter. To treat Jessica's accompanying symptoms of depression, we agreed she would start on an antidepressant. I also encouraged her to make the following behavioral changes:

- Set realistic, attainable goals.
- Break overwhelming tasks down into small steps.
- Focus on one activity or task at a time.
- Acknowledge that everyone makes mistakes.
- Recognize that most mistakes present learning opportunities.
- Confront fears of failure by remaining realistic about possible outcomes.

According to the Mayo Clinic, chronic fatigue syndrome has no cure. Treatment focuses on symptom relief, and the most disruptive or disabling symptoms should be addressed first. In Jessica's case, depression was one of her most significant symptoms, so we started there. A side benefit of the antidepressant she started (Cymbalta) is pain relief. I use it frequently in my patients who have diabetes or chemotherapy-related neuropathies (pins and needles feeling in the feet and hands).

Some people with CFS have difficulty regulating their blood pressure when they change positions. This is called *orthostatic hypotension*. It is normal to have a change in your blood pressure when you move from lying down or sitting to standing. In unaffected people, their autonomic nervous system will automatically adjust. However, for some people with CFS, their autonomic nervous system doesn't get the message, and they will feel dizzy or lightheaded when standing. For those individuals, different medications are available to increase their blood pressure. Sometimes, adding salt to your diet can be helpful.

Energy management (also called pacing) is now emphasized for symptom control. *Pacing* is an individualized approach that monitors energy expenditure to reduce the occurrence, duration, and severity of postexertion malaise. For those suffering from chronic muscle pain, over-the-counter medications such as ibuprofen (for example, Advil and Motrin IB) and naproxen sodium (Aleve) can be helpful. If they are not effective, some medicines used to treat fibromyalgia, like Lyrica, Cymbalta, or Neurontin, may be prescribed.

If you experience sleep deprivation as a result of your symptoms, other symptoms can be more difficult to address. Avoid caffeine or change your bedtime routine. Sleep apnea can be evaluated by a sleep specialist and treated by using a machine that delivers air pressure through a mask while you sleep (CPAP).

Brain fog or cognitive problems associated with CFS are short-term memory issues, distractibility, and feeling overwhelmed by multiple sources of stimulation, such as loud noise, bright lights, or multitasking. These symptoms are likely the result of overtaxing your body and your brain. Interestingly, these symptoms overlap with those of patients who have postconcussion syndrome (PCS), which can occur either soon after or immediately after a head injury. The one big difference is that PCS is directly correlated with a documented head injury. The cause of CFS is still not known. Medication can help treat the cognitive issues associated with CFS. Like patients with attention deficit disorder, the primary symptoms include problems with memory, word-finding, distractibility, and organizational skills. Patients with attention deficit disorder also become extremely fatigued and "crash" when they experience overstimulation. Stimulants like Ritalin, Adderall, and their variants are very useful. They generally work within minutes to an hour and last for several hours. This has the benefit of increasing physical energy and "turning on" your prefrontal cortex, the area of the brain responsible for higher-level cognitive functioning. Such medications also do not accumulate in your blood, so if you experience side effects like decreased appetite or sleep issues, they wear off fairly rapidly.

Tips for Dealing with CFS

- **Push yourself to get moving,** but don't push yourself to do more until you know you're ready. This is what we call reasonable expectations (not perfectionism!). Cognitive difficulties can be caused or exacerbated by overactivity.
- **Take rest breaks and expect some setbacks.** You'll need to experiment to find your current level of tolerance. Just because you take a break doesn't mean you are weak or lazy—it is good for your brain and the rest of your body. Sometimes, short breaks can help with brain fog and muscle fatigue.

- **Realize that exertion comes in all forms.** Avoid significant exercise on a day when you're also going to the grocery store or doing something strenuous. These activities can compound and drain you.
- **Take days off when you need them, but don't give up!** The payoff could be less pain, more energy, and a better quality of life.
- **Practice routine.** Humans and animals do best when their lives are filled with predictable, routine behaviors. If you tend to forget where you place objects, try having a routine to place them in the same place; for example, put your keys in a basket on the table by the door every day. If you travel to work, prepare your lunch and lay out your clothes for the next day at night before you begin your bedtime routine.
- **Use your body's natural rhythms.** Most of us perform better at particular times of day. Some people are better in the early morning, some in the midafternoon. Try to plan your most challenging tasks for the time of day when your energy and concentration are at their peak levels.
- **Let reminders give you a hand up.** Reminders can be your friends. Write out a list of tasks for the day. One of my favorite strategies is to have a whiteboard placed in an area where it cannot be avoided, like the kitchen or in front of your desk. Having that big white board where you can't avoid it seems to make a big difference, and it is far more effective than keeping a list on your phone, which you can easily ignore. Many patients tell me they keep multiple lists and Post-it Notes around the house. While on the surface this sounds admirable, when I ask them if they use them, they almost always say, "No!" So

I subscribe to the "rule of four," which goes like this: On your whiteboard, write down four items you want to accomplish on any given day. A standard reply from my patients is "but I have more than four things I have to do!" I say, "Yes, but if you stick to this method, you will have accomplished twenty tasks by the end of a five-day workweek."

By setting realistic goals this way, you can feel proud that you have accomplished tasks daily instead of berating yourself for not getting enough done.

CHAPTER 13

LIVING IN A FOG OF CONSTANT PAIN: FIBROMYALGIA

*It's every day waking up not knowing
how you're going to feel.*
—LADY GAGA

Dorothy was a thirty-eight-year-old psychologist who was referred to me by her internist. Dorothy dressed flamboyantly and spoke dramatically. Several months before I saw her, she left her husband and took their three-year-old daughter to live with her sister and mother.

Dorothy's internist diagnosed her with fibromyalgia. When she arrived in my office, she described problems with sleep, headaches, daily fatigue, and anxiety. She told me she frequently had dreams of escaping from a dangerous situation. The themes varied from time to time.

I noticed that Dorothy looked around my office often as though she was scanning the environment. When I asked about this, she replied, "Yes, I am always on the lookout for any potentially dangerous situation."

Dorothy told me she believed her father sexually abused her. Her sister, with whom she lived, believed she was as well. According to Dorothy, her nanny found Dorothy's father's underwear in his children's bedroom. Dorothy remembers showering with her father when she was a child, and he used to pretend he was having sex with her stuffed toy horse.

Despite her abusive childhood, Dorothy excelled academically and attended a prestigious university, earning all A's. Even though she achieved academically, she was so depressed in college that she attempted suicide by taking an overdose of Tylenol. After graduation, she worked overseas, and when she returned, she joined a government agency as a specialist. She married a man who was abusive to her and her child, the reason she left the marriage.

When she came to see me, she was under the care of her internist, as well as a rheumatologist who agreed with her diagnosis of fibromyalgia but believed she also had chronic fatigue syndrome. There is a great deal of overlap between these two disorders. The main difference is the predominant symptom of intense muscle and joint pain with fibromyalgia.

Dorothy told me she experienced nightmares, low energy, mental fogginess, and difficulty paying attention and making executive decisions. In the past, she suffered from an eating disorder, which returns from time to time. Her symptoms were affecting her personal and work relationships.

What Is Fibromyalgia?

The concept of fibromyalgia dates back to the early nineteenth century, when physicians described it as *muscular rheumatism*. Fibromyalgia was conceived of as a separate disorder in the 1970s. The American Academy of Rheumatology introduced the first objective criteria, formalizing it as a recognized medical disorder. As is the case with many autoimmune disorders, it is a complex and often misunderstood condition characterized by musculoskeletal pain, tenderness, and a constellation of associated symptoms. Historically, fibromyalgia was frequently met with skepticism within the medical community. This resulted from a lack of knowledge about the disorder, and some practitioners believed it was, you guessed it, "all in the head." Over time, however, advancements in research and a growing body of evidence have uncovered the complex interplay of biological, psychological, and social factors contributing to the syndrome.

What was once regarded as a rare condition is now understood to be a common global health concern. As is often true of autoimmune disorders, more women are diagnosed with this disorder than their male counterparts. It most often occurs in middle age, but cases have also been reported in teens and older adults.

Because fibromyalgia presents with a broad array of symptoms, reaching an accurate diagnosis can be a challenging process. It requires a comprehensive examination of a patient's history, physical examination, and psychosocial factors. The primary symptom of fibromyalgia is widespread chronic muscle and joint pain experienced on both sides of the body. Patients describe the quality of pain as a deep and persistent ache that varies in intensity. Tender points where pressure leads to pain used to be the sole diagnostic criterion, but this is no longer the case due to increased research and knowledge about this disorder.

As you can imagine, patients with fibromyalgia report impaired sleep, initial insomnia (trouble falling asleep) and frequent awakenings. This, unfortunately, leads to a deficit of deep, restorative sleep, a major contributor to the cycle of pain and fatigue. As with CFS, people with fibromyalgia report cognitive problems often referred to as *fibro fog*, along with fatigue and psychiatric symptoms of depression and anxiety.

What Causes Fibromyalgia?

Most medical illnesses are multifactorial. Fibromyalgia is no exception. Research studies have identified specific genetic markers that can make you susceptible to this disorder. The likelihood of inheriting this trait is about 50 percent, so it is common to see fibromyalgia in multiple biological family members. The underlying mechanisms for the genetic predisposition are thought to involve genes responsible for the perception of pain, regulation of your brain chemicals (neurotransmitters), and immune system.

Fibromyalgia is truly a biopsychosocial disorder. Aside from the genetic link, environmental triggers in susceptible people can lead to the onset of this disorder. Specific environmental factors include physical trauma, infections, and stressful life events.

Faulty regulation of neurotransmitters—brain chemicals that are involved in the perception of pain—is a central feature in the development of fibromyalgia. Several neurotransmitters, including serotonin, dopamine, and norepinephrine, are intimately involved in the transmission and perception of pain. Researchers have documented low levels of serotonin in patients who experience chronic pain. One study that looked at female patients with fibromyalgia compared with a healthy control group found that those with the disorder had lower serum levels of serotonin. In addition, they exhibited a positive correlation between their serotonin levels and reported tender touch points.

Norepinephrine plays a significant role in our body's response to stress, and it is dysregulated in patients with fibromyalgia. One study assessed how individuals with fibromyalgia, those with rheumatoid arthritis, and healthy controls perceived pain following a stimulus. All subjects received an injection in their forearms. On one side, the injection was a small amount of norepinephrine; on the other, it was sterile saline. Eighty percent of the fibromyalgia subjects reported pain in response to the norepinephrine injection compared with only 30 percent in the arthritis group and the control group. So, although rheumatoid arthritis is also an autoimmune disorder, there is something clearly different going on with fibromyalgia patients who have an excessive pain experience when provoked by the same stimulus.

Dopamine, another neurotransmitter, is believed to be involved in the mood dysregulation reported by patients with fibromyalgia. One study found that fibromyalgia patients have a disruption in their brain's release of dopamine in response to experimental pain as well as nonpainful stimulation in an area of their brain called the basal ganglia.

Patients with fibromyalgia have abnormalities in their immune systems and, like others with autoimmune disorders, have increased circulating blood levels of inflammatory proteins.

Adverse Life Events

Psychological stressors are social, physical, and environmental factors that challenge an organism's adaptive capabilities and resources. These circumstances represent an extremely wide and varied array of situations including trauma. Trauma can occur at any point in life, but when it happens during childhood or adolescence, its impact is often greater because the central nervous system is still maturing. Research studies show that there is a strong association between childhood trauma and the development of fibromyalgia. In one study, women who reported fibromyalgia symptoms scored higher on a childhood trauma questionnaire compared to their counterparts with different types of pain syndromes or control groups. These findings have been replicated in numerous studies, so trauma in childhood is considered an independent risk factor for all pain syndromes, but more so in patients with fibromyalgia.

Researchers in Spain conducted a yearlong study of eighty-eight women referred from the rheumatology and behavioral health departments at a large hospital in Barcelona. Only participants diagnosed with fibromyalgia were included. Those with major psychiatric diagnoses like schizophrenia and bipolar disorder were excluded. Most of the women were in committed relationships or married, and the average age was fifty-one.

They reported that the most prevalent traumatic events experienced by the participants were physical, sexual, and emotional abuse during childhood and adolescence. There was also a high number of participants who suffered from post-traumatic stress disorder. These findings are very understandable since the participants were chronically and recurrently exposed to different types of stressful events throughout a significant portion of their lives.

Obesity

In many research studies, investigators report that the average body mass index of patients with fibromyalgia is higher than that of their nonaffected counterparts. Recent interest in studying fibromyalgia has thus placed more importance on risk factors for cardiovascular disease such as obesity.

In a 2021 study, researchers found that obesity correlates with pain severity, tender points, stiffness, fatigue, and cognitive problems. Patients with fibromyalgia have more unregulated blood glucose levels and those who practice behaviors to control their weight report an improvement in their overall pain levels.

Management Strategies for Fibromyalgia

Following are practical strategies to help you manage fibromyalgia and support your wellbeing. As with all medical illnesses, treatment should focus on your individual symptoms.

- **Antidepressants** work to modulate pain by regulating the levels of your neurotransmitters that are involved in pain perception. Many antidepressants are available; my preference is to use Cymbalta. It may seem like I prescribe this antidepressant often, and I do. I do not have any financial investment in this choice! The reason I prefer this medication is that it can perform multiple jobs. Cymbalta was initially formulated to treat chronic pain and was preferentially detailed to rheumatologists and physical medicine doctors. After a time, we recognized it as an excellent antidepressant. By using this medication, I can help alleviate the pain associated with this disorder. In addition, depression is prominent in fibromyalgia patients, with 90 percent likely to get depressive symptoms at least once, and 62 to 86 percent at risk of getting major depressive disorder (MDD). Additionally, 40 percent of the time, depression and fibromyalgia occur concurrently.

- **Milnacipran** is not classified as an antidepressant. However, like antidepressants, it impacts brain and plasma levels of serotonin and norepinephrine. In a clinical trial, milnacipran doses of 100 and 200 milligrams per day significantly reduced pain scores compared to a placebo. It not only improves your quality of life but also has few reported side effects. Interestingly, it is approved for depression in parts of Europe, and just like Cymbalta, it helps regulate dysfunctional neurotransmitter transmission.
- Some practitioners use **antiseizure medications**, such as gabapentin, because of their ability to ease neurological pain. They work by reducing nerve activity involved in pain signaling. Unfortunately, one of the side effects is drowsiness.
- **Muscle relaxers**, such as cyclobenzaprine, are often prescribed to reduce muscle spasms. However, many cause sedation and mental confusion, so they are best prescribed at night.

- **Cannabinoids** such as CBD have been investigated as possible treatment options for patients with fibromyalgia. Research findings reported that CBD-rich cannabinoid extract is effective in reducing pain, anxiety, and depression. In most states, you will need a medical marijuana card to access these from a dispensary. However, some online sites, like Charlotte's Web, sell variants of CBD in various forms.
- **Tropisetron** is a medication used to prevent nausea and vomiting in patients undergoing chemotherapy treatment for cancer. It works by blocking the action of serotonin, which binds to nerve cells and shows promise in treating the symptoms of fibromyalgia. For example, research studies show that tropisetron is more effective than a placebo in reducing pain and fatigue. In addition, it improves the overall quality of sleep by decreasing pain and discomfort. In one study, a daily dose of 2 milligrams for five days provided pain relief for up to two months.
- Nonpharmacological treatment, such as **mindfulness-based stress reduction (MBSR)**, improves fibromyalgia symptoms by targeting stress, anxiety, and depression. A recent study in 2022 explored the effectiveness of MBSR as a treatment for fibromyalgia patients. They found positive results, including reductions in pain and fatigue and positive self-reports of overall quality of life.

> **What is MBSR?** The mindfulness-based stress reduction program was first developed in the 1970s by Dr. Jon Kabat-Zinn at the University of Massachusetts Medical School. Although initially designed for stress management, it has evolved to encompass the treatment of various health-related disorders. These include anxiety, depression, skin diseases, pain, immune disorders, hypertension, and diabetes. It employs mindfulness meditation to alleviate suffering associated with physical, psychosomatic, and psychiatric disorders. Over two hundred medical centers worldwide offer MBSR as an alternative treatment option to patients. It is an eight-week course and consists of training for two and a half hours per week with an additional one-day retreat. Participants receive training in formal mindfulness meditation techniques, which include simple stretches and postures.

- **Exercise therapy** that includes aerobic activity and strength training helps treat fibromyalgia symptoms by reducing pain and fatigue and improving physical functioning. **Graded exercise therapy** (GET) involves gradually increasing physical activity levels to improve physical function and relieve pain. It effectively improves physical function but may cause increased pain in some people.
- **Acupuncture** is a traditional Chinese medicine technique that involves the insertion of thin needles into specific points of the body. Only a few studies reported the effectiveness of acupuncture on reducing symptoms of fibromyalgia. However, some patients report its effectiveness in reducing pain and improving the quality of life. More research is needed to

determine the optimal acupuncture points to address, as well as the appropriate length of treatment.

Takeaway Summary for Autoimmune Disorders

Currently, we do not know why some people develop autoimmune disorders while others do not. We do know that autoimmune disorders are being diagnosed on a more frequent basis. According to the National Health Council, "Autoimmune diseases affect approximately 50 million Americans. However, this number is likely underestimated given the complexity of diagnosing these conditions. Even more alarming, autoimmunity is reaching epidemic levels, with some studies estimating an increase of 3 to 12 percent annually." The reasons behind the increasing prevalence of autoimmune diseases are not fully understood. Genetic predispositions, environmental factors—such as pollutants, medications, toxins, and viral infections—and lifestyle factors, including diet, sleep deprivation, stress, and lack of physical activity, all likely play a role.

Awareness and advocacy are crucial in addressing the growing challenge of autoimmune disease. Many patients face significant delays in diagnosis due to vague and overlapping symptoms and the lack of awareness among healthcare providers. Patients with autoimmune disorders visit on average four different providers over four and a half years before receiving a diagnosis and beginning a treatment plan. Increasing awareness about the signs and symptoms of autoimmune diseases can help expedite diagnosis and treatment and improve patient outcomes.

A MENDS Approach for Inflammation and Autoimmune Disorders

- **Medication.** For brain fog associated with autoimmune disorders, I sometimes suggest stimulants, the medicines we prescribe for people with attention deficit disorder. They work quickly, do not build up in your body, and can be used as needed, meaning you do not have to take them daily. Antidepressants can be helpful in some patients with autoimmune disorders, particularly if you are experiencing coexisting depression or anxiety. One antidepressant, Cymbalta, was initially developed as a medication to treat chronic pain. It was later discovered to be an excellent treatment for some patients with depression. In my practice, I use this medication to get a twofold benefit. For those who are experiencing joint pain or muscle aches, as well as a mood or anxiety disorder, this may be an excellent option to treat both symptoms.
- **Exercise.** Exercise benefits patients with autoimmune disorders in several ways. According to a small study published by the National Institute of Health's Intramural Research Program, regular exercise can help with fatigue and overall inflammation in many patients with autoimmune disorders. In their study, female participants with lupus exercised three times per week by walking on a treadmill. At the end of the twelve-week study, the researchers reported delayed fatigue as self-reported by their participants. However, the study went further and found that the parts of their cells called *mitochondria*, which are like little energy sources, actually increased their energy output by the end of the study. The greater a

participant's increase in mitochondrial energy production after twelve weeks of exercise training, the larger their reduction in fatigue symptoms tended to be.

For those with chronic fatigue syndrome, vigorous exercise is not the best choice. Aggressive exercise regimens often lead to worsened symptoms, but maintaining activities that are tolerated is essential to prevent deconditioning. Exercise regimens that start at a very low intensity and gradually increase over time may help improve your long-term function. A side effect of exercise in people who suffer from CFS is, as mentioned earlier, postexertional malaise, which can last for days or weeks after the exertion. There's a sharp increase in symptoms, especially flu-like, following exercise. Moreover, there's an inability to physically repeat the performance the following day. It is vital to find a balance between activity and rest.

Your goal is to remain active but not overdo it. Some exercises that show promise in treating people with CFS are warm-water exercises, like water walking, and Pilates, which is not too aggressive and can help maintain strong muscles, particularly in your core. Other options are tai chi and yoga. Start slowly, observe your symptoms, and find the level of exertion that's right for you.

- **Nutrition.** The medical profession is learning that one of the best ways to reduce inflammation lies not in the medicine cabinet but in the refrigerator. By following an anti-inflammatory diet, you can fight off inflammation for good. To reduce levels of inflammation, aim for an overall healthy diet. A healthy diet is beneficial for reducing the risk of chronic diseases and improving mood and overall quality of life. An anti-inflammatory diet should include these foods:

tomatoes; leafy green vegetables such as spinach, kale, and collards; nuts such as almonds and walnuts; fatty fish such as salmon, mackerel, tuna, and sardines; and fruits such as strawberries, blueberries, cherries, and oranges.

- **Dhyana.** Practicing mindfulness, whether it is meditation, deep breathing exercises, or body scanning, can decrease your stress level and lower the stress hormone cortisol. Increased cortisol output is associated with increased inflammation, a hallmark of autoimmune disorders. Even more interesting, recent studies show that practicing mindfulness can actually change how your genes linked to inflammation and stress are expressed. This means that simple daily practices like meditation could help your body respond better to stress. A study published in the *Journal of High Energy Physics* found that a group of patients with autoimmune liver disease who practiced MBSR with a certified instructor over eight weeks required lower levels of anti-inflammatory medication and had lower blood levels of inflammatory markers.
- **Sleep.** An intricate relationship exists between sleep and autoimmune disorders. Adequate sleep is crucial for maintaining a healthy immune system. Sleep deprivation is associated with increased inflammation, possibly due to increased circulating inflammatory proteins. In addition, sleep deprivation is linked to an increase in chronic pain, which is present in some autoimmune disorders. A study published in *The Lancet* documented the results of a nationwide study from Taiwan that linked non-apnea-related sleep disorders to a higher prevalence of rheumatoid arthritis, lupus, and other autoimmune disorders. The American Academy of Sleep Medicine

(AASM) recommends that adults get at least seven hours of sleep per night regularly. This recommendation is intended to promote optimal health and avoid the health risks of chronic sleep deprivation.

To get better sleep, I recommend that you avoid caffeine or alcohol later in the day. The caffeine will prevent your brain from shutting down adequately and increase your sleep latency. A "nightcap" for sleep is a misnomer. Alcohol may help you fall asleep, but it prevents you from getting into and staying in deep, restorative sleep. You also wake up more frequently.

I also suggest shutting off all your screens—television, computer, and phone—at least sixty minutes before you want to sleep. Your brain is like a big computer, which must shut down in stages. Do not convince yourself you can work on your laptop until 10:00 pm and then try to drift off! Likewise, if you find that you are awake in the middle of the night, fight the urge to jump on your phone.

CHAPTER 14

EPIGENETICS: WHY YOUR DNA IS NOT YOUR DESTINY

Sometimes, when we read about biology, we could be forgiven for thinking that those three letters explain everything.
—NESSA CAREY, The Epigenetics Revolution

Why do identical twins sometimes experience different health outcomes as they age? How is it that a pregnant woman's nutrition can influence her unborn child's future risk of developing certain illnesses? Why are the children of parents who experienced severe trauma more prone to depression decades later? Just how much does our environment shape us?

The answer to all these question is epigenetics. In 1942, biologist Conrad Waddington defined *epigenetics* as the complex interplay between genes inherited from parents and the environment in which one develops. The environment can include the intrauterine environment while one's mother was pregnant, the physical environment after birth, or the psychological environment as one develops.

Epigenetics focuses on how environmental changes can impact your DNA without physically altering it. Mutations occur when your DNA is physically changed, such as by exposure to extreme radiation or chemical toxins. Modifications reflect how your genes are expressed. These modifications can occur in various ways and act as biological switches, turning your genes on or off. This means that while your genetic material itself remains unchanged, the way it functions can be altered. One of the more common epigenetic changes occurs through a process called *methylation*. The addition of this chemical compound can significantly affect the way your genes behave, including altering your risk for developing certain diseases.

Abnormal methylation patterns are associated with several diseases, such as cancer. In these cases, the genes that normally help prevent tumors can become silenced, increasing your risk. Fortunately, many of these changes can be reversed, so scientists are developing new ways to prevent and treat these conditions. That is why I added this chapter to a book about the biopsychosocial view of illness, since these factors can cause epigenetic changes but can also be mitigated through lifestyle changes. I specifically focus on the roles of nutrition, toxic exposures, and the impact of psychological stress.

Prenatal Exposure

When you were a developing fetus, you were exposed to your mother's intrauterine environment. Believe it or not, this may have impacted the likelihood that you would later develop certain diseases. For example, a study published by the Mayo Clinic showed that women who owned pets during their pregnancies gave birth to children who were less likely to develop hypertension when exposed to tobacco smoke or air pollution later in life. The researchers propose that early exposure to germs from domestic animals helps develop the child's immune system.

The well-known Dutch famine birth cohort study was designed to investigate the effects of severe maternal malnutrition during various stages of pregnancy on the likelihood that their offspring would develop certain chronic diseases later in life. The population of Amsterdam experienced severe starvation from 1943 to 1947. On May 10, 1940, the Netherlands was invaded by German troops, which had an immediate impact on the Dutch food supply. Food imports from other countries were no longer possible, and part of the food produced in the Netherlands was sent to Germany. The Dutch registry obtained the birth records of over two thousand children born during those years. Beginning in 1994, the surviving adults were studied about their later development of chronic diseases.

The results showed that prenatal exposure to malnutrition has long-lasting effects on health. The specific effects were linked to when the exposure occurred. For example, the most pronounced effects occurred if the fetus was malnourished during the first trimester, when all major organ systems are formed. The researchers reported that exposure to famine was associated with a higher risk of cardiovascular disease, type 2 diabetes, kidney disease, and respiratory disorders. The sex of the child also made a difference in adulthood. Women who had early exposure had an increased risk of obesity, breast cancer, and mortality. Their male counterparts had more age-related changes on brain MRI scans than expected. Prenatal famine was also associated with increased symptoms of anxiety and depression later in life.

Toxic Exposure

Lead is a naturally occurring toxic metal found in the Earth's crust. Its widespread use has caused extensive environmental contamination, human exposure, and global public health problems. The metal is most often used to manufacture lead-acid batteries for motor vehicles, but it is found in many products, including pigments, paints, stained glass, lead crystal glassware, ammunition, ceramic glazes, jewelry, toys, some traditional cosmetics, and some traditional medicines.

Occupationally, workers in the construction, auto repair, battery manufacturing, and certain mining industries are most at risk for lead exposure. In addition to their exposure, workers in these fields may inadvertently expose their families to this toxin because lead can be tracked onto carpets, floors, and furniture. As in Flint, Michigan, lead pipes can contaminate drinking water.

A very worrisome consequence of this is childhood exposure. Young children are particularly vulnerable to lead poisoning and may absorb up to four to five times as much lead as adults from an ingested dose. Once lead enters your body, it can be distributed to major organs, including your brain, kidneys, liver, and bones. Lead exposure in children can permanently affect their brain development and result in learning issues and behavioral changes. In the most severe cases, it can lead to seizures, coma, or even death. Lead exposure causes a significant disease burden. In 2021, there were over 1 million deaths world-wide caused by lead exposure, primarily due to its effect on the cardiovascular system.

Cigarette smoking can cause epigenetic changes. This is most evident in people who are heavy smokers (smoking twenty or more cigarettes on a daily basis). Smoking-associated DNA methylation alterations in genes can contribute to lung cancer initiation and progression. However, the good news is that if you quit smoking, you can reverse the process and once again develop significant methylation. If you remain abstinent, you can return to levels similar to those of nonsmokers.

It's interesting to note that DNA methylation patterns altered in utero can maintain the altered pattern for years, potentially changing the risk of disease later in life. The same is true for being exposed to secondhand smoke.

Impact of Early Stress

People who experience adverse conditions during childhood show greater vulnerability to psychological illnesses, including depression, post-traumatic stress disorder, bipolar disorder, and anxiety. In addition, traumatic events in childhood are associated with long-term physical health effects. A 2011 study, commonly known as the ACES study, looked at data from a large Canadian Community Health Survey to examine the impact of early childhood trauma on chronic illness in adulthood. They proposed that the development of psychiatric illness in adulthood was a contributing factor to why these participants had higher rates of chronic disease. For example, those with significant psychiatric illnesses like schizophrenia were more likely to live a lifestyle contributing to a higher rate of cardiovascular disease. They were lower in socioeconomic class, more likely to smoke, and ate a fast-food diet high in fat and salt. Those who suffered from mood disorders like depression exercised less, either overate or did not eat a sufficient diet, smoked, and had a higher use of alcohol and other substances. Because of their lower economic status, both groups had less access to adequate medical care.

A more recent review article looked at the impact of stress in children and their later development of inflammatory disorders in adulthood. CRP (C-reactive protein) is a blood marker for inflammation in your body. In one study, British women ages sixty to seventy-nine who were raised in lower socioeconomic environments had higher blood levels of CRP than those raised in more affluent environments. In another study, middle-aged women who had less educated parents had higher levels of CRP compared with those whose parents were more educated. Research shows that children who experience early adversity, whether from psychological or physical trauma or poverty, exhibit a higher level of stress hormones and inflammation when they become adults. Teenagers raised in harsh family environments show higher cytokine (inflammatory protein) production in response to an immune challenge than those raised in a supportive family environment.

Adults with a history of childhood abuse show significantly greater emotional reactivity to daily-life stress compared with those who do not report a history of abuse. Reactions to daily-life stressors are more likely to trigger an inflammatory response. This contributes to many physical diseases, including cardiovascular disease, gastrointestinal disorders, autoimmune disorders, and neurodegenerative disease.

How Can You Modify Your Risk of Disease Impacted by Epigenetics?

Diet. The Mediterranean diet and the DASH diet recommended by the American Heart Association have elements in common. They advocate consuming healthy grains, fruits and vegetables, seafood, and lean meats such as chicken and turkey. Both diets have substantial research to support their benefit in lowering the risk of cardiovascular disease, diabetes, obesity, and inflammatory processes.

A less well-known diet is called the SEAD. Populations in northern Portugal and the northwest Iberian peninsula eat this diet. These regions have some of the largest populations of centenarians. The SEAD contains higher levels of fish and shellfish than the other two. The proteins and omega-3 fatty acids in seafood have a protective effect on cardiovascular health. Interestingly, those who follow the SEAD consume more meat, mostly pork and veal. However, the meat comes from farms where the animals are fed milk and grass—or, in the case of pigs, chestnuts. This type of sustainable farming makes the meat high in healthy protein that is easily digestible. The types of vegetables eaten in the SEAD are different as well. They consume mainly those related to the cabbage family, such as Brussels sprouts, turnips, cauliflower, mustard greens, and rutabaga. Guess what? These vegetables reduce inflammation by limiting the production of inflammatory proteins like cytokines.

Exercise. We all know that exercise is good for our health, and recent research shows that it can impact epigenetic modifications. Scientists in Denmark demonstrated that physical exercise rewires the enhancer sections of our DNA, which are known to be associated with the development of chronic disease. Enhancers regulate which of your genes are switched on or off. For their study, the authors recruited healthy young adults and enrolled them in a six-week endurance exercise program. The researchers obtained a skeletal muscle biopsy before and after the program. After completing the exercise program, they discovered that the skeletal muscle structure of some of the enhancers had been altered. In addition, they found that many enhancers identified in the skeletal muscle are also linked to human diseases. The researchers hypothesized that the beneficial effects of enhancer alterations might also impact distant organs like the brain. In particular, these investigators found that exercise remodeled activity in skeletal muscle that is also linked to cognition.

Exercise improves cognitive function and counteracts age-associated mental decline in older adults. This is related to modifications in the size of the hippocampus, the part of the brain responsible for memory and other executive functions.

Strength training can increase your body's lean mass and decrease insulin resistence. High-intensity intervals can improve your overall metabolism. Even a thirty-minute, moderately intense cycling session can cause epigenetic changes that increase your body's cancer-fighting immune cells. The CDC recommends engaging in at least two and a half hours of aerobic activity weekly and at least two weekly strength workouts for optimal results.

Sleep. Traumatic childhood experiences can trigger epigenetic modifications that not only alter an individual's stress response but can contribute to poor mental health and diseases like cardiovascular discase and high blood pressure. Chronic stress can lead to sleep disturbances, and insufficient sleep is linked to many chronic illnesses, including degenerative brain disorders. Interestingly, the likelihood that you will be prone to sleep deprivation is at least partially genetically linked. Cognitive functions rely on your brain's neuroplasticity—the ability to change and adapt. Most of the harmful epigenetic changes seen in people with sleep deprivation affect genes involved in our twenty-four-hour circadian rhythm and neuroplasticity. For example, people who work night shifts have an altered expression of specific genes involved in their body's internal clock. Current research suggests that most adults must consistently sleep at least seven hours each night to reverse the negative epigenetic changes caused by sleep deprivation.

Social engagement. Humans' ability to form social bonds developed through evolution. In prehistoric times, social groups were essential for survival. Epigenetic changes due to trauma or chronic stress can be an inhibitor to developing social relationships. However, strong social bonds are very important factors in mediating the effects of stress and its adverse effects. Strong social bonds are among the most reliable predictors of self-reported health and happiness. They are also positively related to longevity. Participating in social activities can potentially reverse the effect of epigenetic stress by magnifying the expression of genes associated with resilience and decreasing the expression of negative stress responses.

A large study published in *Brain, Behavior and Immunity* investigated the associations between social relationships and the effects of epigenetic changes in a population of retired adults. They found that those who reported feeling less understood, had few or no people they could rely upon, or felt they could not be truthful and open in their relationships with family or friends had the worst outcomes regarding epigenetic changes. The researchers concluded that it was not just the presence of a social network, but the quality of the relationships formed that had the most beneficial health outcomes in these older adults.

Vitamin supplements. In 2017, researchers at Columbia University reported that B vitamins may play an essential role in reducing the epigenetic effects of air pollution. The World Health Organization estimates that over 90 percent of the world population lives in environments where air quality levels are unhealthy. In this study, investigators administered each participant a B vitamin supplement or placebo. Blood levels of vitamin B were measured in each participant at the beginning and end of the trial. During the experimental phase, air particles from a congested area in downtown Toronto were collected and delivered to the participants through an oxygen-type air mask. The study results showed that the participants who received the B vitamin had a protective effect against the epigenetic change produced by the polluted air. The placebo had no effect.

The science of epigenetics is still in its infancy. However, we know a great deal about how environmental factors can combine with genetics to influence disease development. Let's face it: We don't all win the genetic lottery. However, lifestyle changes can improve how our bodies use our genes through epigenetic modifications.

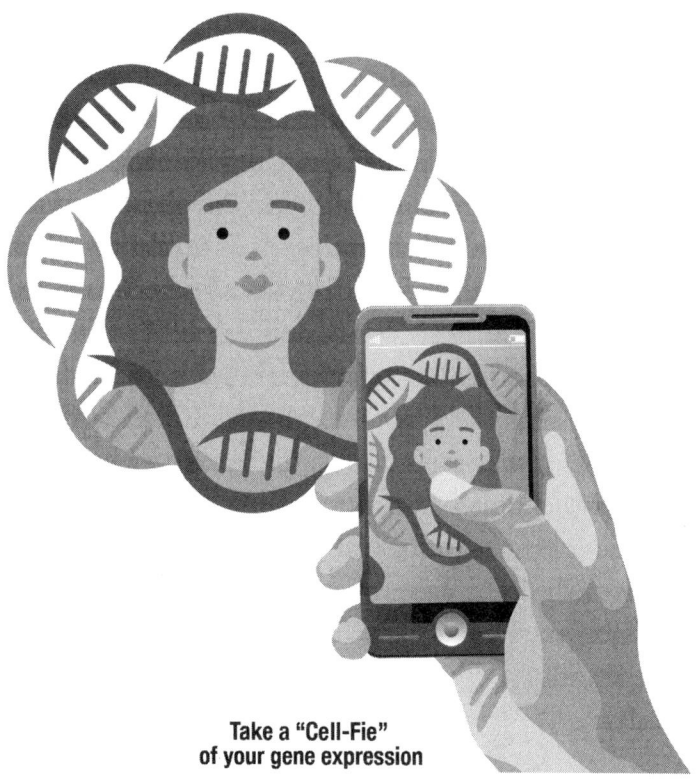

Fig. 14.1 Gene Expressions

EPILOGUE

The idea for this book began almost twenty years ago, fairly early in my career as a psychiatrist. Patients would often ask me if they could read something to learn more about their illness. Sometimes I could offer a reference, but other times, I couldn't find anything appropriate. What I found might have been too technical, or perhaps it wasn't comprehensive enough. At various times, I thought, *Should I write it?* But as with most new challenges, I had my doubts.

My children were still at home, I was running a full-time practice, and I was commuting to Philadelphia every week from my home in Maryland to finish a forensic psychiatry fellowship at the University of Pennsylvania. In short, there just wasn't enough time.

Fast-forward a few decades. My children are out of the house and are successful adults. I still practice full-time but have learned that I enjoy teaching and writing. I have more available time, and finally, three years ago, I thought, *Why not?*

I believe in the quote Hillary Clinton made famous: "It takes a village." However, in my case, it felt more like a universe. There were so many helpful mentors and supporters along the way, and they should all look for their names in the acknowledgment section. I have learned so much in the time since I started writing this. Scientific medical research has changed dramatically since I was a medical student in the late 1980s, and the concept of the mind-body connection has never been more advanced.

Several decades ago, the idea that your physical and mental states are linked was not part of mainstream medicine. But, as hopefully you have learned from reading this book, the concept is not new. Traditional Eastern medicine and the teachings of Hippocrates emphasized that the health of your body and mind are deeply interconnected.

George Engel, the founding father of the biopsychosocial model, was a great admirer of Louis Pasteur, the brilliant French chemist and microbiologist who discovered the principles of vaccination and pasteurization. Pasteur believed in the one-microbe-for-every-illness theory. However, at the end of his life, even he modified his views on disease while studying silkworms. "If I was younger and had to resume my work on silkworms, I'd focus above all on the conditions under which they were raised: [their] living conditions, their food, the temperature in the silkworm sheds and the air inside them—for I am convinced that the worms could be made more resistant to illness if their living conditions were changed."

In the 1960s and 1970s, a cardiologist at Harvard began studying the link between psychosocial stress and blood pressure. In the mid-1970s, a new subspecialty of medicine called *psychoneuroimmunology* published research about how stress and one's emotional state can affect the immune system. A new subspecialty within dermatology called *psychodermatology* studies the link between stress and skin disorders.

Despite this new appreciation of the brain and body in medicine, the phrase "It's all in your head" is still heard far too often. According to one health advocacy site, this dismissive phrase is reported frequently, especially by the 50 million patients who are diagnosed with autoimmune or neurological diseases each year. A study published in *Academic Emergency Medicine* found that women who went to the emergency room with severe stomach pain had to wait almost 33 percent longer than men with the same symptoms. Concerns of female patients are more often seen as less critical than those of their male counterparts. The word *hysteria* actually comes from the ancient Greek and means "uterus." For decades (and sometimes still), the medical community falsely believed that when a woman complained about her health, it was due to hormones or psychological issues.

Now that you have almost finished this book, I hope that you also have a better appreciation for how illness is not just the product of a bacteria, virus, or toxin. As we've learned, illness comes from the complex interplay between your biological, psychological, and social environments. Do not believe medical gaslighters—healthcare providers who you feel are dismissing your concerns or complaints. The signs of gaslighting are not taking you seriously or suggesting your symptoms result from something vague or innocuous, such as "stress," and providers do nothing more about it. Worse, they may send you home without a more informed diagnosis. Aside from feeling dismissed or unheard, these situations can have serious health consequences.

Most doctors go to medical school with good intentions. Gaslighting, as it was first used in film noir, described intentional efforts on the part of an individual to make another doubt their perception of reality. Although surely there are exceptions in medical practice, as there are in other professions, most physicians are not intentionally trying to cause emotional harm by denying patient complaints. However, we are human. We make mistakes and suffer from unconscious bias. For example, heart disease, the number-one killer of women, is often misdiagnosed because it has been regarded as a "male" condition, and women with heart disease frequently present to a doctor's office with symptoms different from those of men. The information we learn in medical school is usually based on research conducted on white males. The data do not translate easily to other populations.

Remember, physicians and other healthcare providers are not omnipotent either. Yes, we train for years to practice our profession, but it is impossible to keep up with all the newly emerging research on every diagnosis. Doctors make mistakes. You are your own best advocate and know your body better than any medical professional. You are paying our fees and have a right to feel respected and have your concerns heard.

So, make sure to have your list of questions handy, especially when you visit a new healthcare provider. Remember, an average office visit is only eighteen minutes long, and you want to have your issues addressed. Bring a trusted friend or relative with you so that you have a second pair of eyes and ears. Do not be afraid to ask about laboratory work or other evaluations that would be helpful in arriving at a diagnosis, or whether you should see a specialist.

You wouldn't hire a contractor without checking their references and reviews, right? So do your homework. You can review the credentials and patient opinions of providers at sites like Healthgrades, WebMD, and Vitals.com.

Finally, bring a copy of this book with you, with your own highlighting if you need to refer to a particular section. Best of luck on your healthcare journey and becoming your own version of a medical Sherlock Holmes!

REFERENCES

Chapter 1: The Biopsychosocial Model ; Why You Should Read This Whole Book

Cheatle, M.D. Biopsychosocial Approach to Assessing and Managing Patients with Chronic Pain. *Med Clin North Am* 100, no. 1 (January 2016): 43–53.

Crouch, T.B., et al. "Pain Rehabilitation's Dual Power: Treatment for Chronic Pain and Prevention of Opioid-Related Risks." *Am Psychol* 75, no. 6 (September 2020): 825–39.

Gatchel, Robert J, et al. "Interdisciplinary Chronic Pain Management: Past, Present, and Future." *American Psychologist*, no. 2 (2014): 119–30.

Levenson, Robert W. "Stress and Illness: A Role for Specific Emotions." *Psychosomatic Medicine*, no. 8 (July 2019): 720–30.

Prego-Domínguez, Jesús, et al. "Socioeconomic Status and Occurrence of Chronic Pain: A Meta-Analysis." *Rheumatology*, no. 3 (December 2020): 1091–105.

Chapter 2: Alexithymia: When There Are No Words

Aust, Sabine, and Malek Bajbouj. "The Role of Early Emotional Neglect in Alexithymia." *The Neuropsychotherapist*, no. 4 (January 2014): 96–97.

Beales, David, and Ros Dalton. "Eating Disordered Patients: Personality, Alexithymia, and Implications for Primary Care." *British Journal of General Practice* (February 2000).

Cerqueira, Andreia, and Telma Catarina Almeida. "Adverse Childhood Experiences: Relationship with Empathy and Alexithymia." *Journal of Child & Adolescent Trauma*, no. 3 (February 2023): 559–68.

Cohen, Karen, et al. "Is Alexithymia Related to Psychosomatic Disorder and Somatizing?" *Journal of Psychosomatic Research*, no. 2 (February 1994): 119–27.

Di Tella, Marialaura, and Lorys Castelli. "Alexithymia in Chronic Pain Disorders." *Current Rheumatology Reports*, no. 7 (May 2016).

Freiherr von Schoenhueb, D., B. Boecking, and B. Mazurek. "Alexithymia in Patients with Somatization Difficulties and Tinnitus-Related Distress: A Systematic Review." *J Clin Med.* no. 21 (October 29, 2023): 6828.

Kano, Michiko, and Shin Fukudo. "The Alexithymic Brain: The Neural Pathways Linking Alexithymia to Physical Disorders." *BioPsychoSocial Medicine*, no. 1 (2013): 1.

Kojima, Masayo. "Alexithymia as a Prognostic Risk Factor for Health Problems: A Brief Review of Epidemiological Studies." *BioPsychoSocial Medicine*, no. 1 (2012): 21.

Kooiman, Cornelis G., et al. "Is Alexithymia a Risk Factor for Unexplained Physical Symptoms in General Medical Outpatients?" *Psychosomatic Medicine*, no. 6 (November 2000): 768–78.

Larsen, Junilla K., et al. "Cognitive and Emotional Characteristics of Alexithymia." *Journal of Psychosomatic Research*, no. 6 (June 2003): 533–41.

Lumley, Mark A., et al. "The Assessment of Alexithymia in Medical Settings: Implications for Understanding and Treating Health Problems." *Journal of Personality Assessment*, no. 3 (November 2007): 230–46.

Nakao, Mutsuhiro, and Takeaki Takeuchi. "Alexithymia and Somatosensory Amplification Link Perceived Psychosocial Stress and Somatic Symptoms in Outpatients with Psychosomatic Illness." *Journal of Clinical Medicine*, no. 5 (May 2018): 112.

Sancassiani, Federica, et al. "Why Is It Important to Assess and Treat Alexithymia in the Cardiologic Field? An Overview of the Literature." *Clinical Practice and Epidemiology in Mental Health*, no. 1 (August 2023).

Smakowski, Abigail, et al. "Psychological Risk Factors of Somatic Symptom Disorder: A Systematic Review and Meta-Analysis of Cross-Sectional and Longitudinal Studies." *Journal of Psychosomatic Research* (June 2024): 111608.

Xu, Pengfei, et al. "Structure of the Alexithymic Brain: A Parametric Coordinate-Based Meta-Analysis." *Neuroscience and Biobehavioral Reviews* (April 2018): 50–55.

Chapter 3: Your Achy-Breaky Heart: The Role of Stress in Heart Disease

Chams, Sana, et al. "Zumba-Induced Takotsubo Cardiomyopathy: A Case Report." *Journal of Medical Case Reports*, no. 1 (June 2018).

Cuffee, Yendelela, et al. "Psychosocial Risk Factors for Hypertension: An Update of the Literature." *Current Hypertension Reports*, no. 10 (August 2014).

Goldstein, Jill M., et al. "Sex Differences in Major Depression and Comorbidity of Cardiometabolic Disorders: Impact of Prenatal Stress and Immune Exposures." *Neuropsychopharmacology*, no. 1 (July 2018): 59–70.

Kivimäki, Mika, and Andrew Steptoe. "Effects of Stress on the Development and Progression of Cardiovascular Disease." *Nature Reviews Cardiology*, no. 4 (December 2017): 215–29.

Landa, Eric, et al. "A Broken Heart: A Case of Takotsubo Cardiomyopathy." *Cureus* (November 2021).

Morera, Luis Pedro, et al. "Stress, Dietary Patterns and Cardiovascular Disease: A Mini-Review." *Frontiers in Neuroscience* (November 2019).

Nayeri, Arash, et al. "Psychiatric Illness in Takotsubo (Stress) Cardiomyopathy: A Review." *Psychosomatics*, no. 3 (May 2018): 220–26.

Osborne, Michael T., et al. "Disentangling the Links Between Psychosocial Stress and Cardiovascular Disease." *Circulation: Cardiovascular Imaging*, no. 8 (August 2020).

Spruill, Tanya M. "Chronic Psychosocial Stress and Hypertension." *Current Hypertension Reports*, no. 1 (January 2010): 10–16.

Steptoe, Andrew, et al. "Introduction to Cardiovascular Disease, Stress and Adaptation," 1–14. In *Stress and Cardiovascular Disease*. London: Springer, 2011.

Tawakol, Ahmed, et al. "Relation Between Resting Amygdalar Activity and Cardiovascular Events: A Longitudinal and Cohort Study." *The Lancet*, no. 10071 (February 2017): 834–45.

Trudel-Fitzgerald, Claudia, et al. "Dysregulated Blood Pressure: Can Regulating Emotions Help?" *Current Hypertension Reports*, no. 12 (October 2015).

Chapter 4: What's Good for the Heart Is Good for the Brain: The Link Between Depression and Heart Disease

Amare, A. T., et al. "The Genetic Overlap Between Mood Disorders and Cardiometabolic Diseases: A Systematic Review of Genome Wide and Candidate Gene Studies." *Translational Psychiatry*, no. 1 (January 2017): e1007.

Ananthakrishnan, Ashwin, et al. "Association Between Depressive Symptoms and Incidence of Crohn's Disease and Ulcerative Colitis: Results from the Nurses' Health Study." *Clinical Gastroenterology Hepatology* (January 2013).

Boehm, Julia, and Laura Kub. "The Heart's Content: The Association Between Positive Psychological Well-Being and Cardiovascular Health." *Psychological Bulletin* (2012).

Davies, Simon J. C., et al. "Treatment of Anxiety and Depressive Disorders in Patients with Cardiovascular Disease." *BMJ*, no. 7445 (April 2004): 939–43.

Deschênes S. S., R. J. Burns, and N. Schmitz. "Depressive Symptoms and Sleep Problems as Risk Factors for Heart Disease: A Prospective Community Study." *Epidemiol Psychiatr Sci.* 29 (August 20, 2019): e50.

References

Goldstein, Jill M., et al. "Sex Differences in Major Depression and Comorbidity of Cardiometabolic Disorders: Impact of Prenatal Stress and Immune Exposures." *Neuropsychopharmacology*, no. 1 (July 2018): 59–70.

Jeyanantham, Kishaan, et al. "Effects of Cognitive Behavioural Therapy for Depression in Heart Failure Patients: A Systematic Review and Meta-Analysis." *Heart Failure Reviews*, no. 6 (July 2017): 731–41.

Kwapong, Yaa A., et al. "Association of Depression and Poor Mental Health with Cardiovascular Disease and Suboptimal Cardiovascular Health Among Young Adults in the United States." *Journal of the American Heart Association*, no. 3 (February 2023).

LaChance, Laura R., and D. Ramsey. "Antidepressant Foods: An Evidence-Based Nutrient Profiling System for Depression." *World Journal of Psychiatry*, no. 3 (September 2018): 97–104.

Lee, Su Nam, et al. "Impacts of Gender and Lifestyle on the Association Between Depressive Symptoms and Cardiovascular Disease Risk in the UK Biobank." *Scientific Reports*, no. 1 (July 2023).

Li, Xinzhong, et al. "Cardiovascular Disease and Depression: A Narrative Review." *Frontiers in Cardiovascular Medicine* (November 2023).

Lu, Qi, et al. "Depressive Symptoms, Lifestyle Behaviors, and Risk of Cardiovascular Disease and Mortality in Individuals of Different Socioeconomic Status: A Prospective Cohort Study." *Journal of Affective Disorders* (February 2024): 345–51.

Mingjing, Shao, et al. "Depression and Cardiovascular Disease: Shared Molecular Mechanisms and Clinical Implications." *Psychiatry Research* (March 2020).

Pizzagalli, Diego, and Angela Roberts. "Prefrontal Cortex and Depression." *Neuropsychopharmacology* (January 2022).

Seldenrijk, Adrie, et al. "Depression, Anxiety and 6-Year Risk of Cardiovascular Disease." *Journal of Psychosomatic Research*, no. 2 (February 2015): 123–29.

Shiga, Tsuyoshi. "Depression and Cardiovascular Diseases." *Journal of Cardiology* (May 2023).

Whooley, Mary A., et al. "Depression and Inflammation in Patients with Coronary Heart Disease: Findings from the Heart and Soul Study." *Biological Psychiatry*, no. 4 (August 2007): 314–20.

Zambrano, Juliana, et al. "Psychiatric and Psychological Interventions for Depression in Patients with Heart Disease: A Scoping Review." *Journal of the American Heart Association*, no. 22 (November 2020).

Chapter 5: Butterflies in Your Stomach and Other Gut Phenomena

Ananthakrishnan, Ashwin N. "Environmental Risk Factors for Inflammatory Bowel Diseases: A Review." *Digestive Diseases and Sciences*, no. 2 (September 2014): 290–98.

Bray, Nicola A., et al. "Evaluation of a Multidisciplinary Integrated Treatment Approach Versus Standard Model of Care for Functional Gastrointestinal Disorders (FGIDS): A Matched Cohort Study." *Digestive Diseases and Sciences*, no. 12 (April 2022): 5593–601.

Chitkara, Denesh K., et al. "Early Life Risk Factors That Contribute to Irritable Bowel Syndrome in Adults: A Systematic Review." *The American Journal of Gastroenterology*, no. 3 (March 2008): 765–74.

"How Exercise Can Lead to a Healthy Gut." January 26, 2024. https://health.clevelandclinic.org/gut-health-workout.

Hsu, Wen-Yu, et al. "Escitalopram for Psychogenic Nausea and Vomiting: A Report of Two Cases." *Journal of the Formosan Medical Association*, no. 1 (January 2011): 62–66.

Keefer, Laurie, and Sunanda Kane. "Considering the Bidirectional Pathways Between Depression and IBD: Recommendations for Comprehensive IBD Care." *Gastroenterology and Hepatology* (March 2017).

Kelly, John R., et al. "Breaking Down the Barriers: The Gut Microbiome, Intestinal Permeability and Stress-Related Psychiatric Disorders." *Frontiers in Cellular Neuroscience* (October 2015).

References

Lee, Sang-Yeol, et al. "A Study of Psychological Factors Associated with Functional Gastrointestinal Disorders and Use of Health Care." *Clinical Psychopharmacology and Neuroscience*, no. 4 (November 2020): 580–86.

McGuinness, Amelia J., et al. "Mood Disorders: The Gut Bacteriome and Beyond." *Biological Psychiatry*, no. 4 (February 2024): 319–28.

Muraoka, M., et al. "Psychogenic Vomiting: The Relation Between Patterns of Vomiting and Psychiatric Diagnoses." *Gut*, no. 5 (May 1990): 526–28.

Ohlsson Gustafsson, Lavant Suneson, Brundin Westrin, et al. "Leaky Gut Biomarkers in Depression and Suicidal Behavior." *Acta Psychiatrica Scandinavica*, no. 139 (2019): 185–93.

Olden, Kevin, and Pavan Chepyala. "Functional Nausea and Vomiting." *Gastroenterology and Hepatology* (February 2008).

Patel, Amit, et al. "Sensory Neuromodulators in Functional Nausea and Vomiting: Predictors of Response." *Postgraduate Medical Journal*, no. 1049 (October 2012): 131–36.

Peirce, Jason M., and Karina Alviña. "The Role of Inflammation and the Gut Microbiome in Depression and Anxiety." *Journal of Neuroscience Research*, no. 10 (May 2019): 1223–41.

Rathour, Deepak, et al. "Role of Gut Microbiota in Depression: Understanding Molecular Pathways, Recent Research, and Future Direction." *Behavioural Brain Research* (January 2023): 114081.

Smith, Robert P., et al. "Gut Microbiome Diversity Is Associated with Sleep Physiology in Humans." *PLOS One* (October 2019): e0222394.

Sun, Yue, et al. "Stress Triggers Flare of Inflammatory Bowel Disease in Children and Adults." *Frontiers in Pediatrics* (October 2019).

Turpin, William. "Environmental Factors Associated with Risk of Crohn's Disease Development in a Prospective Cohort of Healthy First-Degree Relatives of Crohn's Disease Patients." *Digestive Disease Week* (2022).

Whitfield, K. Lynette, and Robert J. Shulman. "Treatment Options for Functional Gastrointestinal Disorders: From Empiric to Complementary Approaches." *Pediatric Annals*, no. 5 (May 2009): 288–94.

Xiong, Ruo-Gu, et al. "The Role of Gut Microbiota in Anxiety, Depression, and Other Mental Disorders as Well as the Protective Effects of Dietary Components." *Nutrients*, no. 14 (July 2023): 3258.

Zingone, Fabiana, et al. "Psychological Morbidity of Celiac Disease: A Review of the Literature." *United European Gastroenterology Journal*, no. 2 (April 2015): 136–45.

Chapter 6: Is Your Stomach Depressed? The Link Between Your Gut and Mood

Alli, Sauliha R., et al. "The Gut Microbiome in Depression and Potential Benefit of Prebiotics, Probiotics and Synbiotics: A Systematic Review of Clinical Trials and Observational Studies." *International Journal of Molecular Sciences*, no. 9 (April 2022): 4494.

Busby, Eleanor, et al. "Review Mood Disorders and Gluten: It's Not All in Your Mind! A Systematic Review with Meta-Analysis." *Nutrients* (October 2018).

Chinna Meyyappan, Arthi, et al. "Effect of Fecal Microbiota Transplant on Symptoms of Psychiatric Disorders: A Systematic Review." *BMC Psychiatry*, no. 1 (June 2020).

Doll, Jessica, et al. "Fecal Microbiota Transplantation (FMT) as an Adjunctive Therapy for Depression—Case Report." *Frontiers in Psychiatry* (February 2022).

Gao, Jie, et al. "Probiotics for the Treatment of Depression and Its Comorbidities: A Systemic Review." *Frontiers in Cellular and Infection Microbiology* (April 2023).

Green, Jessica E., et al. "Safety and Feasibility of Faecal Microbiota Transplant for Major Depressive Disorder: Study Protocol for a Pilot Randomised Controlled Trial." *Pilot and Feasibility Studies*, no. 1 (January 2023).

"How Exercise Can Lead to a Healthy Gut." January 26, 2024. https://health.clevelandclinic.org/gut-health-workout.

Huang, Cancan, et al. "Safety and Efficacy of Fecal Microbiota Transplantation for Treatment of Systemic Lupus Erythematosus: An EXPLORER Trial." *Journal of Autoimmunity* (June 2022): 102844.

Huang, Ting-Ting, et al. "Current Understanding of Gut Microbiota in Mood Disorders: An Update of Human Studies." *Frontiers in Genetics* (February 2019).

Keefer, Laurie, and Sunanda Kane. "Considering the Bidirectional Pathways Between Depression and IBD: Recommendations for Comprehensive IBD Care." *Gastroenterology and Hepatology* (March 2017).

Limbana, Therese, et al. "Gut Microbiome and Depression: How Microbes Affect the Way We Think." *Cureus* (August 2020).

Liu, Lu, and Gang Zhu. "Gut-Brain Axis and Mood Disorder." *Frontiers in Psychiatry* (May 2018).

Macedo, Danielle, et al. "Antidepressants, Antimicrobials or Both? Gut Microbiota Dysbiosis in Depression and Possible Implications of the Antimicrobial Effects of Antidepressant Drugs for Antidepressant Effectiveness." *Journal of Affective Disorders* (January 2017): 22–32.

McGuinness, Amelia J., et al. "Mood Disorders: The Gut Bacteriome and Beyond." *Biological Psychiatry*, no. 4 (February 2024): 319–28.

Molska, Marta, et al. "The Influence of Intestinal Microbiota on BDNF Levels." *Nutrients*, no. 17 (August 2024): 2891.

Petra, Anastasia I., et al. "Gut-Microbiota-Brain Axis and Its Effect on Neuropsychiatric Disorders with Suspected Immune Dysregulation." *Clinical Therapeutics*, no. 5 (May 2015): 984–95.

Rathour, Deepak, et al. "Role of Gut Microbiota in Depression: Understanding Molecular Pathways, Recent Research, and Future Direction." *Behavioural Brain Research* (January 2023): 114081.

Rutsch, Andrina, et al. "The Gut-Brain Axis: How Microbiota and Host Inflammasome Influence Brain Physiology and Pathology." *Frontiers in Immunology* (December 2020).

Smith, Robert P., et al. "Gut Microbiome Diversity Is Associated with Sleep Physiology in Humans." *PLOS One* (October 2019): e0222394.

Chapter 7: Can COVID Cause Psychiatric Symptoms

Benzakour, Lamyae, and Guido Bondolfi. "Update of the Potential Treatments for Psychiatric and Neuropsychiatric Symptoms in the

Context of the Post-COVID-19 Condition: Still a Lot of Suffering and Many More Things to Learn." *Trauma Care*, no. 2 (March 2022): 131–50.

Bushi, Ganesh, et al. "Postural Orthostatic Tachycardia Syndrome After COVID-19 Vaccination: A Systematic Review." *BMC Cardiovascular Disorders*, no. 1 (November 2024).

Ceban, Felicia, et al. "Registered Clinical Trials Investigating Treatment of Long COVID: A Scoping Review and Recommendations for Research." *Infectious Diseases*, no. 7 (March 2022): 467–77.

Efstathiou, Vasiliki, et al. "Long COVID and Neuropsychiatric Manifestations (Review)." *Experimental and Therapeutic Medicine*, no. 5 (April 2022).

Hunter, Philip. "Viral Diseases and the Brain." *EMBO Reports*, no. 1 (November 2021).

Kubota, T., et al. "Neuropsychiatric Aspects of Long COVID: A Comprehensive Review." *Psychiatry and Clinical Neurosciences* (2022).

Mallick, Deobrat, et al. "COVID-19 Induced Postural Orthostatic Tachycardia Syndrome (POTS): A Review." *Cureus* (March 2023).

Pahwa, Roma, et al. "Chronic Inflammation." *StatPearls Publishing* (August 2023).

Paunescu, Ramona, et al. "Acute and Long-Term Psychiatric Symptoms Associated with COVID19 (Review)." *Biomed Reports* (November 2022).

Stefanou, Maria-Ioanna, et al. "Neurological Manifestations of Long-COVID Syndrome: A Narrative Review." *Therapeutic Advances in Chronic Disease* (January 2022).

Trachman, Susan. "Chronic Inflammation Is Linked to Psychiatric Disorders." *Psychology Today* (July 5, 2023).

Tsuchida, Tomoya, et al. "Treatment of Long COVID Complicated by Postural Orthostatic Tachycardia Syndrome—Case Series Research." *Journal of General and Family Medicine*, no. 1 (December 2023): 53–61.

"Update of the Potential Treatments for Psychiatric and Neuropsychiatric Symptoms in the Context of the Post-COVID-19 Condition: Still a Lot of Suffering and Many More Things to Learn." *Trauma Care*, no. 2 (March 2022): 131–50.

Zawilska, Jolanta B., and Katarzyna Kuczyńska. "Psychiatric and Neurological Complications of Long COVID." *Journal of Psychiatric Research* (December 2022): 349–60.

Zhang K, K., X. Zhou, H. Liu, and K. Hashimoto. "Treatment Concerns for Psychiatric Symptoms in Patients with COVID-19 With or Without Psychiatric Disorders." *Br J Psychiatry* 217, no. 1 (July 2020): 351.

Chapter 8: Lyme Disease: The Great Imitator

Baker, Phillip J. "Is It Possible to Make a Correct Diagnosis of Lyme Disease on Symptoms Alone? Review of Key Issues and Public Health Implications." *The American Journal of Medicine*, no. 10 (October 2019): 1148–52.

Biniaz-Harris, Nicholas, et al. "Neuropsychiatric Lyme Disease and Vagus Nerve Stimulation." *Antibiotics*, no. 9 (August 2023): 1347.

Coiffier, Guillaume, and Pierre Tattevin. "Lyme Disease: 'End of the Debate'?" *Joint Bone Spine*, no. 4 (July 2021): 105181.

Csallner, Gisela, et al. "Patients with 'Organically Unexplained Symptoms' Presenting to a Borreliosis Clinic: Clinical and Psychobehavioral Characteristics and Quality of Life." *Psychosomatics* (2013).

Fallon, Brian A., et al. "Lyme Borreliosis and Associations with Mental Disorders and Suicidal Behavior: A Nationwide Danish Cohort Study." *American Journal of Psychiatry*, no. 10 (October 2021): 921–31.

Rebman, Alison W., and John N. Aucott. "Post-Treatment Lyme Disease as a Model for Persistent Symptoms in Lyme Disease." *Frontiers in Medicine* (February 2020).

Ścieszka, Joanna, et al. "Post–Lyme Disease Syndrome." *Rheumatology*, no. 1 (February 2015): 46–48.

Van Hout, Marie Claire. "The Controversies, Challenges and Complexities of Lyme Disease: A Narrative Review." *Journal of Pharmacy & Pharmaceutical Sciences* (November 2018): 429–36.

Wong, Katelyn, et al. "A Review of Posttreatment Lyme Disease Syndrome and Chronic Lyme Disease for the Practicing Immunologist." *Clinical Reviews in Allergy and Immunology* (2022).

Chapter 9: Epstein-Barr Virus: Not Just the Kissing Disease

Gold J. E., R. A. Okyay, W. E. Licht, and D. J. Hurley. "Investigation of Long COVID Prevalence and Its Relationship to Epstein-Barr Virus Reactivation." *Pathogens*. 10, no. 6 (June 17, 2021): 763.

Harley, John B., et al. "Transcription Factors Operate Across Disease Loci, with EBNA2 Implicated in Autoimmunity." *Nature Genetics*, no. 5 (April 2018): 699–707.

Vindegaard, Nina, et al. "Infectious Mononucleosis as a Risk Factor for Depression: A Nationwide Cohort Study." *Brain, Behavior, and Immunity* (May 2021): 259–65.

Chapter 10: Inflammation and Brain Function

Beatriz Currier, M., and Charles B. Nemeroff. "Inflammation and Mood Disorders: Proinflammatory Cytokines and the Pathogenesis of Depression." *Anti-Inflammatory & Anti-Allergy Agents in Medicinal Chemistry*, no. 3 (September 2010): 212–20.

Black, David S., and George M. Slavich. "Mindfulness Meditation and the Immune System: A Systematic Review of Randomized Controlled Trials." *Annals of the New York Academy of Sciences* (January 2016): 13–24.

Haroon, Ebrahim, et al. "Inflammation, Glutamate, and Glia: A Trio of Trouble in Mood Disorders." *Neuropsychopharmacology*, no. 1 (September 2016): 193–215.

Jones, Brett D. M., et al. "Inflammation as a Treatment Target in Mood Disorders: Review." *British Journal of Psychiatry Open*, no. 4 (June 2020).

Miller, Andrew, and Charles Raison. "The Role of Inflammation in Depression: From Evolutionary Imperative to Modern Treatment Target." *Nature Review Immunology* (January 2016).

Chapter 11: When the Body Attacks Itself: The Mysteries of Autoimmune Disorders and Related Phenomena

Alrabadi, Leina S., et al. "Mindfulness-Based Stress Reduction May Decrease Stress, Disease Activity, and Inflammatory Cytokine Levels in Patients with Autoimmune Hepatitis." *JHEP Reports*, no. 5 (May 2022): 100450.

Bertagnolli, Monica. "Study Offers New Clues to Why Most People with Autoimmune Diseases Are Women." National Institutes of Health (blog), February 15, 2024.

Dolgin, Elie. "Why Autoimmune Disease Is More Common in Women: X Chromosome Holds Clues." *Nature*, no. 7999 (February 2024): 466.

Itoh, Yuichiro, et al. "The X-Linked Histone Demethylase Kdm6a in CD4+ T Lymphocytes Modulates Autoimmunity." *Journal of Clinical Investigation*, no. 9 (August 2019): 3852–63.

Kronzer, Vanessa L., et al. "Why Women Have More Autoimmune Diseases Than Men: An Evolutionary Perspective." *Evolutionary Applications*, no. 3 (December 2020): 629–33.

Levy, Brandon. "Role of Sleep Deprivation in Immune-Related Disease Risk and Outcomes." NIH Intramural Research Program. February 7, 2023.

Liu, Yanjun, and Xiangqi Tang. "Depressive Syndromes in Autoimmune Disorders of the Nervous System: Prevalence, Etiology, and Influence." *Frontiers in Psychiatry* (September 2018).

Moore, Breshay. "A Major Health Crisis: The Alarming Rise of Autoimmune Disease." National Health Council (blog). March 28, 2024.

Niazi A. K., and S. K. Niazi. "Mindfulness-Based Stress Reduction: A Non-Pharmacological pproach for hronic Illnesses." *N Am J Med Sci* 3, no. 1 (January 2011): 20–23.

Rosenblat, Joshua D., et al. "Inflamed Moods: A Review of the Interactions Between Inflammation and Mood Disorders." *Progress in Neuro-Psychopharmacology and Biological Psychiatry* (August 2014): 23–34.

Sarwar, Sobia, et al. "Neuropsychiatric Systemic Lupus Erythematosus: A 2021 Update on Diagnosis, Management, and Current Challenges." *Cureus* (September 2021).

Sciarra, Francesca, et al. "Gender-Specific Impact of Sex Hormones on the Immune System." *International Journal of Molecular Sciences*, no. 7 (March 2023): 6302.

Song, Huan, et al. "Association of Stress-Related Disorders with Subsequent Autoimmune Disease." *JAMA* (June 2018): 2388.

Trachman, Susan. "Why Are Autoimmune Disorders More Common in Women?" *Psychology Today* (February 21, 2024).

Weiss, David B., et al. "Psychiatric Manifestations of Autoimmune Disorders." *Current Treatment Options in Neurology*, no. 5 (October 2005): 413–17.

Chapter 12: When You're Running on Empty: Chronic Fatigue Syndrome

Arron, Hayley E., et al. "Myalgic Encephalomyelitis/Chronic Fatigue Syndrome: The Biology of a Neglected Disease." *Frontiers in Immunology* (June 2024).

Graves, B. Sue, et al. "Chronic Fatigue Syndrome: Diagnosis, Treatment, and Future Direction." *Cureus* (October 2024).

Noor, Nazir, et al. "A Comprehensive Update of the Current Understanding of Chronic Fatigue Syndrome." *Anesthesiology and Pain Medicine*, no. 3 (June 2021).

Trachman, Susan B. "She's Not Imagining It: The Continuing Medical Dismissal of Women | Psychology Today." Psychology Today, https://www.psychologytoday.com/us/blog/its-not-just-inyour-head/202507/shes-not-imagining-it-the-continuing-medical-dismissal-of. Accessed 23 Nov. 2025.

Walitt, Brian, et al. "Deep Phenotyping of Post-Infectious Myalgic Encephalomyelitis/Chronic Fatigue Syndrome." *Nature Communications*, no. 1 (February 2024).

Chapter 13: Living in a Fog of Constant Pain: Fibromyalgia

Al Sharie, S., et al. "Unraveling the Complex Web of Fibromyalgia: A Narrative Review." *Medicina* (Kaunas). 60, no. 2 (February 4, 2024): 272.

Creed, Francis. "A Review of the Incidence and Risk Factors for Fibromyalgia and Chronic Widespread Pain in Population-Based Studies." *Pain*, no. 6 (February 2020): 1169–76.

English, Clayton, et al. "Milnacipran (Savella), a Treatment Option for Fibromyalgia." *Pharmacy and Therapeutics* (2010).

Galvez-Sánchez, Carmen M., et al. "Psychological Impact of Fibromyalgia: Current Perspectives." *Psychology Research and Behavior Management* (February 2019): 117–27.

Gardoki-Souto, Itxaso, et al. "Prevalence and Characterization of Psychological Trauma in Patients with Fibromyalgia: A Cross-Sectional Study." *Pain Research and Management* (November 2022): 1–16.

Lourenço, Sara, et al. "Gender and Psychosocial Context as Determinants of Fibromyalgia Symptoms (Fibromyalgia Research Criteria) in Young Adults from the General Population." *Rheumatology*, no. 10 (May 2015): 1806–15.

Ram, Pothuri R., et al. "Beyond the Pain: A Systematic Narrative Review of the Latest Advancements in Fibromyalgia Treatment." *Cureus* (October 2023).

Chapter 14: Epigenetics: Why Your DNA Is Not Your Destiny

Abraham, M. J., et al. "Restoring Epigenetic Reprogramming with Diet and Exercise to Improve Health-Related Metabolic Diseases." *Biomolecules*. 13, no. 2 (February 7, 2023): 318.

Alegría-Torres, Jorge Alejandro, et al. "Epigenetics and Lifestyle." *Epigenomics* (August 2017).

Bakulski, K. M., et al. "DNA Methylation Signature of Smoking in Lung Cancer Is Enriched for Exposure Signatures in Newborn and Adult Blood." *Scientific Reports*, no. 1 (March 2019).

Bleker, Laura S., et al. "Cohort Profile: The Dutch Famine Birth Cohort (DFBC)—a Prospective Birth Cohort Study in the Netherlands." *BMJ Open* (March 2021).

Danieli, Maria Giovanna, et al. "Exposome: Epigenetics and Autoimmune Diseases." *Autoimmunity Reviews*, no. 6 (June 2024): 103584.

Fagundes, Christopher P., and Baldwin Way. "Early-Life Stress and Adult Inflammation." *Current Directions in Psychological Science*, no. 4 (August 2014): 277–83.

Farrell, Allison K., et al. "The Impact of Stress at Different Life Stages on Physical Health and the Buffering Effects of Maternal Sensitivity." *Health Psychology*, no. 1 (January 2017): 35–44.

Farsetti, Antonella, et al. "How Epigenetics Impacts on Human Diseases." *European Journal of Internal Medicine* (August 2023): 15–22.

Friso, Simonetta, et al. "Vitamins and Epigenetics." *Molecular Nutrition* (2020): 633–50.

Ho, S. M., et al. "Environmental Epigenetics and Its Implication on Disease Risk and Health Outcomes." *ILAR Journal*, no. 3–4 (December 2012): 289–305.

Jiang, Xia, and Lars Alfredsson. "Modifiable Environmental Exposure and Risk of Arthritis—Current Evidence from Genetic Studies." *Arthritis Research Therapy*, no. 1 (June 2020).

Lorenzo, Paula M., et al. "Epigenetic Effects of Healthy Foods and Lifestyle Habits from the Southern European Atlantic Diet Pattern: A Narrative Review." *Advances in Nutrition*, no. 5 (September 2022): 1725–47.

Mock, Steven E., and Susan M. Arai. "Childhood Trauma and Chronic Illness in Adulthood: Mental Health and Socioeconomic Status as Explanatory Factors and Buffers." *Frontiers in Psychology* (2011).

Rentscher, Kelly E., et al. "Social Relationships and Epigenetic Aging in Older Adulthood: Results from the Health and Retirement Study." *Brain, Behavior, and Immunity* (November 2023): 349–59.

Roseboom, Tessa J., et al. "Effects of Prenatal Exposure to the Dutch Famine on Adult Disease in Later Life: An Overview." *Twin Research*, no. 5 (October 2001): 293–98.

Thakur, Chitra, et al. "Epigenetics and Environment in Breast Cancer: New Paradigms for Anti-Cancer Therapies." *Frontiers in Oncology* (September 2022).

Thumfart, Kristina M., et al. "Epigenetics of Childhood Trauma: Long-Term Sequelae and Potential for Treatment." *Neuroscience & Biobehavioral Reviews* (January 2022): 1049–66.

Yehuda, Rachel. "How Parents' Trauma Leaves Biological Traces in Children." *Scientific American*, July 2022.

Yu, Xinyang, et al. "Cancer Epigenetics: From Laboratory Studies and Clinical Trials to Precision Medicine." *Cell Death Discovery*, no. 1 (January 2024).

Zhong, Jia, et al. "B Vitamins Attenuate the Epigenetic Effects of Ambient Fine Particles in a Pilot Human Intervention Trial." *Proceedings of the National Academy of Sciences*, no. 13 (March 2017): 3503–8.

Epilogue

Chen, Esther H., et al. "Gender Disparity in Analgesic Treatment of Emergency Department Patients with Acute Abdominal Pain." *Academic Emergency Medicine* (March 2008): 414–18.

Neprash, Hannah T., et al. "Measuring Primary Care Exam Length Using Electronic Health Record Data." *Medical Care*, no. 1 (November 2020): 62–66.

Trachman, Susan. "Patients with Unexplained Symptoms and Medical Gaslighting." *Psychology Today* (March 2, 2023).

Figures and Tables

Fig. 3.1 Similarities Between an Octopus Pot and Imaging from a Patient with Takotsubo's Cardiomyopathy from *American Journal of Case Reports 14* (November 2013): 494–97.

Fig. 3.2 The Amygdala Hijack
Adapted from: https://wholeminds.org.uk/whole-minds-blog/stress-and-how-to-manage-it-agpxn

Fig. 3.3 Composition of the Human Nervous System
Adapted from: https://edupub.org/2022/01/16/the-nervous-system

Fig. 3.4 The Relationship Between Well-Being and Cardiovascular Health
Adapted from: *J Am Coll Cardiol* 72, no. 12 (September 18, 2018): 1382–96.

Fig. 4.1 Pathways for Depression and CVD
From: Depression and Cardiovascular Disease: Shared Molecular Mechanisms and Clinical Implications. *Psychiatry Research* 28.

Fig. 6.1 Multiple Variables Influence the Gut Environment
Adapted from: 'Influence of Intestinal Microbiota on BDNF Levels.' *Nutrients*. 16, no. 17 (August 29, 2024): 2891.

Fig. 6.2. Comparison Between a Healthy Versus Damaged Gut Membrane
Adapted from: Biomaterial-Tight Junction Interaction and Potential Impacts. *Journal of Materials Chemistry*, Issue 41, 2019.

Fig. 8.1 Classic Lyme Bull's-Eye Lesion
From https://www.cdc.gov/lyme/signs-symptoms/lyme-disease-rashes

Fig. 9.1 The Effect of Stress on Health and Athletic Performance
Adapted from: M. R. Salleh, "Life Event, Stress, and Illness," *Malaysian Journal of Medical Sciences* 15, no. 4 (October 2008): 9–18.

Fig. 10.1 The Inflammatory Response
Adapted from https://quizlet.com/191191830/immune-system-frq-flas-cards

Fig. 10.2 Autoimmune Disorders in Various Organ Systems
From: https://www.dhdmed.com/blogs/blog-posts/what-is-autoimmune-disease

Table. 11.1 Manifestations of Central and Peripheral Nervous System Disorders. From Sarwar et al. *Cureus 13, no. 9 (2021)*: e17969. DOI 10.7759/cureus.17969

RESOURCES AND FURTHER READING

Section I: New Insights into The Mind-Body Connection

Bolton D, Gillett G. The Biopsychosocial Model of Health and Disease: New Philosophical and Scientific Developments [Internet]. Cham (CH): Palgrave Pivot; 2019. Chapter 1, The Biopsychosocial Model 40 Years On. 2019 Mar 29. Available from: https://www.ncbi.nlm.nih.gov/books/NBK552030

The Alexithymia Awareness Network: https://alexithymiaawarenessnetwork.org/resources

The Alexithymia Workbook: Overcome Emotional Blindness and Enrich Your Emotional Connections by Wagner Philips.

Section II: Cardiovascular Disease

Recovery & Support for Takotsubo Syndrome https://nyulangone.org/conditions/takotsubo-syndrome/support

In Search of Coronary-Prone Behavior: Beyond Type A by Aron Wolfe Siegman and Theodore Dembroski.

The DASH Diet: https://www.mayoclinic.org/healthy-lifestyle/nutrition-and-healthy-eating/in-depth/dash-diet

The Mediterranean Diet: https://mediterraneanplan.com/quiz

Box Breathing video: https://www.youtube.com/watch?v=oN8xV3Kb5-Q

Section III: Your Two Brains

Cognitive Behavioral Therapy: Feeling Good: The New Mood Therapy by David D. Burns, MD. https://www.amazon.com/Feeling-Good-New-Mood-Therapy

Celiac Disease Foundation: https://celiac.org

Celiac Friendly Restaurants: National Celiac Association https://national-celiac.org/restaurants-dining-out

Anti-Inflammatory Diet: https://www.hopkinsmedicine.org/health/wellness-and-prevention/anti-inflammatory-diet

Section IV: Sneaky Diseases and Psychiatric Symptoms

AAPM&R Long COVID Consensus Guidance Statements: https://www.aapmr.org/members-publications/newsroom/member-news/2021/12/14/aapm-r-long-covid-consensus-guidance-statements

Mindfulness-Based Stress Reduction Program: https://palousemindfulness.com

Amy Tan Suffers Lyme Disease: A Genius Mind Goes Missing: https://youtu.be/YMVbh03kAbY?si=A5Q8LjjYQOGPzKZq.

Section V: Your Brain on Fire

The Hygiene Hypothesis, Johns Hopkins Bloomberg School of Public Health: https://publichealth.jhu.edu/2022/is-the-hygiene-hypothesis-true

Brain on Fire: My Month of Madness by Susannah Cahalan. https://www.amazon.com/Brain-Fire-My-Month-Madness

Jon Kabat-Zinn website: https://jonkabat-zinn.com

The SEAD Diet: Carballo-Casla A, Stefler D, Ortolá R, Chen Y, Knuppel A, Kubinova R, Pajak A, Rodríguez-Artalejo F, Brunner EJ, Bobak M. The Southern European Atlantic diet and all-cause and cause-specific mortality: a European multicohort study. *Eur J Prev Cardiol.* 2024 Feb 15;31(3):358-367.

ABOUT THE AUTHOR

Dr. Susan Trachman is a recurring contributor for the blog "It's Not Just in Your Head" on *Psychology Today*, where her articles are designated as essential reading and published on the front page. She receives frequent requests for media interviews and has been featured in *Washingtonian Magazine, Psychiatry Advisor.com, Mental—The Podcast to Destigmatize Mental Health,* and *Wellness Radio with Dr. J.*

Dr. Trachman is a psychiatrist with over thirty years of clinical and academic experience. She is double board-certified in adult psychiatry and forensic psychiatry. She graduated from the University of Texas McGovern Medical School, where she was inducted into Alpha Omega Alpha, the medical honor society. She was also awarded the Janet Glasgow Memorial Award for academic scholarship.

After graduation, Dr. Trachman completed an internship and residency in psychiatry at the George Washington Medical Center in Washington, DC. For her fourth year, she was selected to be the Chief Resident, supervising medical students and junior physicians.

Dr. Trachman was selected for the competitive fellowship in psychosomatic medicine at Georgetown University Medical Center. During her fellowship, she consulted on hundreds of patients at a major teaching hospital, many of whom presented with medically unexplained symptoms.

She was invited to join the teaching faculty, where she contributed to the education of medical students, residents, and fellows from three local medical schools. Dr. Trachman remains on the teaching faculty at George Washington University Medical School and Virginia Commonwealth Medical School.

In 1990, Dr. Trachman completed her second fellowship in forensic psychiatry at the University of Pennsylvania. She consults with attorneys, human relations professionals, and organizations regarding questions of psychological damages and workplace harassment.

Dr. Trachman is published in peer-reviewed journals including *Psychosomatics* and *Postgraduate Obstetrics and Gynecology*. She authored a book chapter entitled "Post Traumatic Stress Disorder in Litigation" published in *Malingering, Lies and Junk Science in the Courtroom*, by Jack Kitaeff, and had a feature article, "The Dual Role Dilemma" published in both the *Journal of the Arlington Bar Association* and *The Fairfax Bar Journal*.

Dr. Trachman is regularly included in *Washingtonian Magazine's* Best Doctors in Washington issues and *Northern Virginia Magazine's* Best Doctors based on votes from her peers. Based on patient reviews, she received the Compassionate Doctor Award.

Dr. Trachman lives in Virginia with her domestic zoo, which includes two dogs and two cats. When not in the office, you can find her harvesting her vegetable garden or hiking in the woods with her two canine companions.